LIGHTEN UP!

Tija Petrovich

DELICIOUS
HOMESTYLE
COOKING FOR
LOWFAT LIVING

PRIMA PUBLISHING

PRIMA PUBLISHING and colophon are trademarks of Prima Communications, Inc.

Library of Congress Cataloging-in-Publication Data

Petrovich, Tija.
    Lighten up! : delicious homestyle cooking for lowfat living / by Tija Petrovich.
        p.   cm.
    Includes index.
    ISBN 0-7615-0299-8
    1. Low-fat diet—Recipes.   I. Title.
RM237.7.P48   1992
641.5'638—dc20   95-42184
                                               CIP

96 97 98 99 00 AA 10 9 8 7 6 5 4 3 2 1

Printed in the United States of America

Nutritional Breakdowns
A per serving nutritional breakdown is provided for each recipe. If a range is given for an ingredient amount, the breakdown is based on the smaller number. If a range is given for servings, the breakdown is based on the larger number. If a choice of ingredients is given in an ingredient listing, the breakdown is calculated using the first choice. Nutritional content may vary depending on the specific brands or types of ingredients used.

How to Order
Single copies may be ordered from Prima Publishing, P.O. Box 1260BK, Rocklin, CA 95677; telephone (916) 632-4400. Quantity discounts are also available. On your letterhead, include information concerning the intended use of the books and the number of books you wish to purchase.

To our courage and commitment
to make changes and to the happier,
healthier lifestyles that follow.

CONTENTS

Delicious dressings, spreads, dips, sauces, and salsas.
Exciting flavors to spread around. Rediscover
natural fruit toppings, gravy, pesto, and much more.

Fresh fruits, pancakes, hot cereals, hash browns,
and sausage are *some* of the eye-opening suggestions
for a super breakfast or special brunch.

Home-baked aromas in *your* kitchen. Effortless,
wonderful ways to bake your own breads, rolls,
muffins, and memories.

Definitely *not* rabbit food! Well balanced, satisfying
salads for quick luncheons or leisurely dinners.

Lighter side soups and cold weather warmers.
Experience these harmonious flavors as first
courses or as delicious full meals.

ACKNOWLEDGMENTS

I appreciate the unconditional love, understanding, and support of my loved ones, clients, and those whose lives have touched mine. I thank you for your unique gifts and inspirations.

To my "tasters" for their loving honesty.

Special thanks to Sandy Hogan for her support, personal faith, and push that helped me to realize a possibility.

INTRODUCTION

Are you storing excess, unwanted body fat? Have you dieted or altered your natural nutritional requirements and achieved frustrating results—namely, starvation and weight gain? Are you tired of no-fat and no-flavor foods?

This book is designed as a basic source of information, recipes and guidelines for anyone seeking to improve their eating behavior, reduce excess fat levels, or create nutritional lifestyle changes. My focus is to introduce delicious and appealing lowfat recipes to support these changes and ensure your lowfat fitness!

While fat is an essential nutrient, too much fat can be detrimental to your health. Your personal body fat level is a result of a combined number of influences. Elevated fat levels can be linked to high dietary fat intake, excessive carbohydrate consumption, unhealthy stress behaviors, and your own genetic structure. The storage of fat is merely an energy storing process inherited from our primitive ancestors. The body initially created the fat cell to store large amounts of calories in a small space. These calories were then used during lengthy starvation periods. From these primitive ancestors, your body inherited an internal weight regulating system. This system keeps you at a set level of body fat determined by the dietary information that you provide your body. When you diet, you send the same starvation information to your system that the primitive man sent to his. Your body registers a decrease in calorie intake as a threat to your life and responds by slowing down its metabolic rate and storing fat as fuel for your survival. Unlike our active ancestors, in the western world we are generally semi-sedentary societies. We rarely experience true starvation or utilize our extra stored fat as fuel. Dieting to lose this stored fat only increases hunger, signaling our body to store *more* fat. Our body then becomes accustomed to this new level of fat and seeks to maintain it.

The answer to lowering excess body fat is to change behaviors that influence your system to store high levels of fat. Adopt healthy nutritional lifestyle behaviors that signal your system to safely decrease your fat level. Well-balanced, lowfat nutrition, coupled with fat burning physical activities can lower set levels of fat. Aerobic activities utilize fat stored for energy. The aerobic benefit is not the burning of calories but rather stimulating fat metabolism for hours after your aerobic activity is completed. A moderate 30-minute session, three times a week, will aid in fat loss. As in any new change, regular exercise may take a while to become a permanent habit. Vary your aerobic activities to avoid boredom (cycling, swimming, tennis, brisk walking or jumping rope are good aerobic choices). Learn to value your health, not thinness.

To keep you inspired and committed to your new lifestyle, this book is filled with delicious lowfat recipes from my own kitchen. Learn how to improve your cooking techniques, make informed food and fat choices, and enjoy your own home cooking. Most of the recipes in this book do not contain added oils or fats. As a result, you are able to select your personal oil preferences. Please read the *Guidelines* section and the information provided in the *In Preparation* section carefully for information regarding nutritional and essential fats.

Finally, start slowly, develop reasonable and obtainable goals and enjoy a healthy lifestyle!

Step-by-Step Tips to Success ∂◎

1. **Eat a broad variety of beneficial and nutritive food.**

    Provide your body with the food it requires. Maintain a daily dietary ratio of 65% carbohydrate, 20–25% protein, and 10–15% fat. Carbohydrate choices should include *both* starchy (glucose) carbohydrates such as whole grains, potatoes, rice, and squash, and fibrous (cleansing) carbohydrates such as asparagus, broccoli, cauliflower, cabbage, and spinach. Excessive intake of starchy carbohydrates will increase blood sugar (glucose) levels, triggering hunger, and unused carbo-hydrates will store in your body as fat! Excessive intake of fibrous carbohydrates can create inadequate nutrient diges-tion due to the quick passage and elimination of these foods. Moderation is the key here. Protein sources may include chicken, turkey, egg whites, and fish in 3–4 oz portions.

2. Reduce your daily fat intake.

Learn to distinguish "good fat" from "bad fat." Structure your fat intake (10–15%) to small amounts of monounsaturated and polyunsaturated fats and small amounts of some cold-water fish. Measure your oil use in teaspoon amounts and your cold-water fish in 3–4 oz portions. This will keep your focus on the nutritional and therapeutic sources of essential fatty acids needed for a healthy diet.

Choosing an oil can be tricky, depending upon your intended use. A fresh flax or wheat germ oil is a good choice to lightly sprinkle over cold foods and salads. For light cooking and lower baking temperatures (below 325°F) choose *unrefined,* true cold-pressed oils. These oils include olive, pumpkin seed, soy, and walnut oils, and are dark in color. If canola oil is your unsaturated choice, I urge caution and suggest your own re-search. Canola oils have been known to contain toxic erucic acid, linked to heart disease. For baking above 325°F, a *refined* soy or walnut oil will perform the best. Refined oils, such as those found in most grocery stores, have low nutritional value but are more stable to light, heat, and air. Use all oils sparingly. Store all types of oils in a refrigerator to avoid spoilage.

Avoid highly processed store oils and foods containing satu-rated fats such as coconut oil, palm oil, beef, pork, visible animal fat and skin, and whole fat dairy products. Even a 2% milk can draw over 33% of its calories from fat!

For a healthy, complete diet, do *not* reduce your fat intake below 10%. This can be considered unhealthy and neglectful of your body's nutritional needs. Use limited amounts of "good fats" to maintain proper body functions, provide essential nutritional fat levels, and help prolong your body's digestive process to create a "full" sensation.

3. **Eliminate junk foods and lower your sugar intake.**

   Junk foods are a major source of hidden fats, sugars, and excessive calories. Consumption of processed sugars causes an increase in appetite and a rise in blood sugar levels, which in turn are linked to energy and mood changes. Artificial sugars have also been known to increase appetite. Learn to choose appropriate, wholesome snacks such as fruits, potatoes, or vegetables to maintain a steady blood sugar level.

4. **Eat 5 to 6 small meals each day.**

   Eat quality foods at regular and consistent intervals. Do not tax your system by forcing it to digest huge quantities of food! You will find that your body *cannot* fully digest large meals, leaving you with extra bulk to store as fat. Listen to your natural hunger drive. When you are hungry, eat. When you are full, stop. Eating smaller, more frequent meals helps burn calories more efficiently and maintains energy levels.

5. **Drink plenty of water.**

   Water helps with fat metabolism. A lack of water may cause your natural waste system to slow down and your body fat will increase. Drink at least 8–10 glasses a day. Even when you're not thirsty, your body can be dehydrated. Dehydration can often be misinterpreted as hunger. Don't miss your body's natural signal for water. Satisfy a true thirst with water—not coffee, tea, milk, juice, or other liquids. These only contain extra calories and do not satisfy your body's thirst.

6. **Begin an aerobic exercise program.**

   Choose an aerobic activity that you enjoy (biking, tennis, swimming, swift walking). Ask friends to join you, and exercise *three* times per week, resting a day between sessions to recover. Start out slowly and comfortably, training 8–10 minutes. Work your way up to 30 minutes each time. The goal in aerobic exercise is to stimulate fat metabolism, not burn calories. Utilize the fat your body has stored for energy. A leaner lifestyle change should be slow and consistent. Start out gradually and enjoy the many benefits that exercise can provide.

7. Read those labels.

Take a few moments to become nutritionally informed. Purchase products that have true nutrition value versus those whose calories come mostly from fats and sugars. Remember that the first ingredients listed are those that the product contains in greater portions. Labeling is not proportioned equally. For example, a product with three ingredients can have a 50%, 48%, and 1% breakdown, a 90%, 9%, and 1% breakdown, or any other combination. Compare fat, sugar, and calorie intake per serving of a product. If a portion seems extremely small, it could be high in fat, sugar, and calories.

Beware of catch phrases such as "sugar-free," "lower in fat," "dietetic," or "high in fiber." Sugar comes in many forms (sucrose, fructose, dextrose, sorbitol, xylose, lactose, corn syrup, honey, molasses, and many more), so choose carefully. Since sugars can be listed individually, check the label to ensure it only appears once. Be aware that some "lowfat" products are high in sugar to make them tastefully attractive. "Dietetic" does not mean low calorie, just sweetened with a sugar replacer. "Dietetic low sugar" products can be high in fat. When choosing "lower in fat" products, such as "fat reduced" meats, you could still be getting well over half your calories from fat! "High fiber" products may also be saturated with fats and sugars. Demand the most nutrition for your calorie and learn to decipher food labels.

8. Overall, use moderation!

Making personal changes can be frustrating. Start slowly and gradually. Don't force yourself into nutrition perfection. Developing healthy patterns should be educational and enjoyable. It could take months or years to change a lifetime of poor nutritional patterns or periods of dieting. I believe that eating is a behavioral issue and good patterns can be developed over time, not overnight. Start with your own personal nutrition awareness. Respond to your body's true physiological hunger, not to psychological influences. Outline a percentage of body fat appropriate for you, and start a step-by-step modification program allowing you freedom to change. Don't envision your choices as black and white; just adapt to each new situation. Learn to substitute your foods and balance your behaviors! Great health is a "long term" choice.

Inside Information: Reading Beyond Labels ᔪ

Nutrition labeling can fool even a health-conscious shopper. Emotional catch phrases such as "no cholesterol," "light," "lowfat," or "% fat free" appear on a wide variety of food products. However, this type of labeling can be misleading, and may be more designed to sell the product by playing on a consumer's emotions than it is to provide any type of useful information.

Often product labels do not provide the information necessary to make a proper nutritional choice. For example, "no cholesterol" products can still be high in saturated, artery-clogging fats. Remember that *only* animal products contain actual cholesterol. Another example is the word "light," which can refer simply to a product's color or texture and not to its nutritional value. Finally, products "lower in fat" and "% fat free" can still be high in fat calories. The percent of fat is based on product *weight*, not on calories!

You *can* find useful information on a food's label if you know how to determine the food's nutritional value. Below is an example of nutrition labeling from a carton of 2% milk:

Serving size:	One cup (8 oz)
Servings per container:	4
Calories:	136
Protein:	10 g
Carbohydrate:	13 g
Fat:	5 g
Sodium:	143 mg

To determine the nutritional value, you'll need to calculate the percentage of calories from carbohydrates, protein, and fat. Remember that one gram (g) of carbohydrate or protein contains 4 calories. One gram of fat contains 9 calories. An 8 oz serving of 2% milk contains 136 calories. So:

Calorie total =   136/serving

To calculate % of calories from carbohydrate:

13 g × 4 calories/g =   52 calories
52 ÷ 136 (total calories) = .38 or 38% carbohydrates

To calculate % of calories from protein:

10 g × 4 calories/g =   40 calories
40 ÷ 136 (total calories) = .29 or 29% protein

To calculate % of calories from fat:

5 g × 9 calories/g =   45 calories
45 ÷ 136 (total calories) = .33 or 33% fat

One third of this product is fat.

In this book, I've chosen to display my recipe information using some of the same nutrition labeling most widely available. My emphasis is based on the fat gram to help you quickly calculate your fat intake. The number of recommended fat grams per serving of food varies, depending upon the use of the food itself (dinner, snack, beverage, etc.). Calculate the percentage of fat calories in all your foods by reading nutritional labels or by using a food composition table. As some meals are higher or lower in fat than others, structure your daily fat intake to reflect your overall dietary food consumption.

Before you start cooking, it is important that you read the glossary on pages 201 to 210. It defines healthy foods that will help you understand how to *Lighten Up* for good!

Chapter 1

AT THE TOP

At the Top

DRESSINGS
Creamy Curry Dressing
Creamy Italian Dressing
Honey Mustard Dressing
Cucumber Dressing
Orange Poppy Seed Dressing
Fresh Veggie Dip

SALSAS
Island Salsa
South Border Salsa
Tex Mex Salsa

SAUCES
Basic White Sauce
Beef Gravy
Chunky Pasta Sauce
Dijon Curry Sauce
Jamaican Sweet and Sour Sauce
My Best Barbecue Sauce
Pinch-Hitting Pesto
Tartar Sauce

JUST FOR FUN
Citrus Sauce
Cranberry "Plus" Sauce
Creamy Select Sauce
Natural Fruit Topping
Warm Vanilla Sauce

SPREADS
Black Bean Spread
Cinnamon Spread
Cream Cheese Stand-In
Mock Mayo
Sour Cream Replacer

🐚 CREAMY CURRY DRESSING

Total yield: 24 servings or 1 ¹/₂ C
Serving size: 1 T
Each serving provides:
Calories: 12
Protein: 1 gram
Fat: trace (1.2 grams total/recipe)
Carbohydrate: 1.89 grams

²/₃ C 1 percent cottage cheese

¹/₄ C plain nonfat yogurt

¹/₄ C nonfat milk

2 T honey

1 tsp curry powder (to taste)

¹/₈ tsp ground ginger

1. Combine all ingredients in blender; blend until smooth.
2. Chill and serve.

Tops a variety of salads, vegetables, or fruits.

✂ CREAMY ITALIAN DRESSING

Total yield: 20 servings or 1 1/4 C
Serving size: 1 T
Each serving provides:
Calories: 11
Protein: 1.5 grams
Fat: trace (2.5 grams total/recipe)
Carbohydrate: 0.97 gram

1 C percent cottage cheese

2 T 1 1/2 percent buttermilk

2 T plain nonfat yogurt

1 tsp lemon juice

1/4 tsp garlic powder

1/4 tsp onion powder
(no salt added)

1/8 tsp crushed oregano

1/8 tsp crushed basil

1/8 tsp crushed parsley

1. Combine all ingredients in blender; blend until smooth.
2. Chill and serve.

ᘓ HONEY MUSTARD DRESSING

Total yield: 16 servings or 1 C
Serving size: 1 T
Each serving provides:
Calories: 9
Protein: 0.9 gram
Fat: trace (0.7 gram total/recipe)
Carbohydrate: 1.26 grams

1 C plain nonfat yogurt

1 T Dijon mustard

2 tsp honey (to taste)

1. Whisk ingredients together in small bowl.
2. Chill and serve.

℞ CUCUMBER DRESSING

Total yield: 24 servings or 1 ¹/₂ C
Serving size: 1 T
Each serving provides:
Calories: 5
Protein: 0.6 gram
Fat: 0
Carbohydrate: 0.65 gram

1 large cucumber (1 C grated)

1 C plain nonfat yogurt

¹/₂ tsp lemon juice

¹/₂ tsp fresh parsley, minced

pinch garlic powder

pinch pepper

1. Peel and section cucumber lengthwise and remove seeds.

2. Using a cheese grater, grate or shred cucumber.

3. Pat dry with a paper towel.

4. Place shredded cucumber and remaining ingredients in a blender; blend until smooth.

5. Chill and serve.

⟨⟨ ORANGE POPPY SEED DRESSING

Total yield: 18 servings or 1 ¹/₈ C
Serving size: 1 T
Each serving provides:
Calories: 11
Protein: 0.7 gram
Fat: trace (1 gram total/recipe)
Carbohydrate: 1.93 grams

1 C plain nonfat yogurt

1 T honey

1 T orange juice concentrate

1 tsp poppy seeds

1 tsp grated orange peel

1. Combine all ingredients in small mixing bowl.
2. Blend until smooth, either by hand or using an electric mixer.
3. Chill and serve.

Serve over your favorite salad.

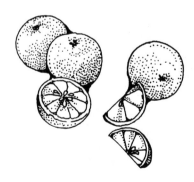

✑ FRESH VEGGIE DIP

Total yield: 16 servings or 1 C
Serving size: 1 T
Each serving provides:
Calories: 10
Protein: 1.2 grams
Fat: trace (1 gram total/recipe)
Carbohydrate: 1.16 grams

$^1/_2$ C 1 percent cottage cheese

$^1/_2$ C plain nonfat yogurt

2 tsp chopped green onion

2 tsp fresh snipped parsley

1 tsp white wine vinegar

$^1/_2$ tsp chopped fresh cilantro
(or fresh mint)

$^1/_4$ tsp garlic powder

pinch ground white pepper

1. Combine all ingredients in blender; blend until smooth.
2. Chill at least one hour and serve.

Serve with a colorful veggie tray, or spoon inside a hot baked potato.

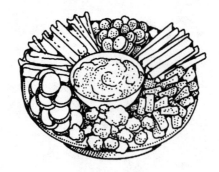

AT THE TOP

🕊 ISLAND SALSA

Total yield: 8 servings or 2 C
Serving size: ¹/₄ C
Each serving provides:
Calories: 34
Protein: 0.5 gram
Fat: trace (0.7 gram total/recipe)
Carbohydrate: 7.8 grams

1 C chopped pineapple tidbits
(fresh or water-packed)

1 C fresh papaya (approximately
1 medium papaya, seeded,
peeled, and chopped)

¹/₄ C diced shallots

1 T lime juice

1 tsp jalapeño pepper, finely chopped

1 tsp granulated fructose

¹/₄ tsp fresh ginger, grated

1 ¹/₂ T fresh mint or cilantro, minced

1. Combine all ingredients in a glass bowl and mix well.

2. For a smooth-pouring salsa, blend 5–10 seconds in blender
before chilling (salsa should be chunky).

3. Cover and chill 2–3 hours before serving.

Serve over blackened fish for a zesty entree.

❧ SOUTH BORDER SALSA

Total yield: 16 servings or 4 C
Serving size: ¹/₄ C
Each serving provides:
Calories: 10
Protein: 0.33 gram
Fat: trace (1.2 grams total/recipe)
Carbohydrate: 2 grams

4 large tomatoes, peeled and chopped

³/₄ C white onion, diced (1 medium)

¹/₄ C fresh cilantro, minced

2 T lemon juice

2 T canned green chilies, diced

1 clove garlic, pressed

¹/₄ tsp ground cumin

pinch ground red pepper

1. In a large glass bowl, combine all ingredients.
2. For a smooth-pouring salsa, blend 5–10 seconds in blender before chilling (salsa should be chunky).
3. Cover and refrigerate one hour.

Serve this salsa with chicken or fish, or spooned inside a hot baked potato.

ᏧᎷ TEX MEX SALSA

Total yield: 9 servings or 2 ¹/₄ C
Serving size: ¹/₄ C
Each serving provides:
Calories: 16
Protein: 0.57 gram
Fat: trace (0.8 gram total/recipe)
Carbohydrate: 3.23 grams

1 C red onion, diced

1 C red bell pepper, diced

1 C natural salsa (sugar- and oil-free)

¹/₄ tsp each: ground cumin, paprika,
garlic powder, dried oregano, dried thyme

pinch cayenne

1. Combine all ingredients in a small mixing bowl.
2. For a smooth-pouring salsa, blend 5–10 seconds before chilling (salsa should be chunky).
3. Mix well and chill.

This can be used as a spicy baste when broiling your favorite poultry or fish.

⚞ BASIC WHITE SAUCE

Total yield: 16 servings or 1 C
Serving size: 1 T
Each serving provides:
Calories: 9
Protein: 0.5 gram
Fat: trace (0.7 gram total/recipe)
Carbohydrate: 1.65 grams

1 C nonfat milk

1 T cornstarch

1 1/2 tsp flour

1 T dry Butter Buds

pepper to taste

1. In a saucepan, whisk together milk, cornstarch, and flour.

2. Stir over medium heat to thicken.

3. Remove from heat; add remaining ingredients and stir.

4. Serve immediately.

To create an herb sauce for fish or chicken, in Step 3 add:
2 tsp fresh, snipped herbs (basil, dill, or thyme)
1 tsp parsley
1 tsp chives

ᑕ BEEF GRAVY

Total yield: 8 servings or 2 C
Serving size: ¹/₄ C
Each serving provides:
Calories: 14
Protein: 0.8 gram
Fat: trace (1 gram total/recipe)
Carbohydrate: 2.41 grams

2 C beef bouillon, cold
(low-salt and defatted if possible)

1 ¹/₂ T cornstarch

1 T flour

2 tsp dry onion soup mix

pepper to taste

1. In a small saucepan, whisk together cold bouillon, cornstarch and flour.

2. Stir in remaining ingredients.

3. Cook over medium heat, stirring constantly with whisk until mixture thickens.

4. Serve immediately.

⊘ CHUNKY PASTA SAUCE

Total yield: 6 servings or 6 C
Serving size: 1 C
Each serving provides:
Calories: 97
Protein: 4.2 grams
Fat: 0.4 gram
Carbohydrate: 19.15 grams

2 (15-ounce) cans chunky tomato sauce

1 (4-ounce) can sliced mushrooms, drained

2 C eggplant, chopped into 1-inch cubes

1 medium red bell pepper, chopped

1 medium yellow bell pepper, chopped

$^3/_4$ C sweet onion, chopped

3 medium cloves garlic, diced

2 T dry red wine (optional)

1 tsp white wine vinegar

1 tsp granulated fructose

2 bay leaves, whole

$^1/_2$ tsp dry sweet basil

$^1/_4$ tsp each rubbed sage and dry rosemary

$^1/_8$ tsp crushed thyme

pinch of black pepper

1. In a large saucepan or small dutch oven, combine all ingredients and bring to boil.

2. Reduce heat to simmer; cover and cook over low heat for 1 hour, stirring occasionally.

3. Turn off heat; let stand 1 $^1/_2$ hours.

4. Remove bay leaves; rewarm to serve.

ᐠ DIJON CURRY SAUCE

Total yield: 16 servings or 1 C
Serving size: 1 T
Each serving provides:
Calories: 9
Protein: 0.5 gram
Fat: trace (0.6 gram total/recipe)
Carbohydrate: 1.66 grams

1 C nonfat milk

1 T cornstarch

1 ¹/₂ tsp flour

1 tsp Dijon mustard

³/₄ tsp curry powder

1. In a small saucepan, whisk together milk, cornstarch, and flour.

2. Heat until thick and bubbly, stirring with a wire whisk.

3. Remove from heat, stir in curry powder and mustard.

Spice that rice! Serve over brown rice or chicken.

⊙ JAMAICAN SWEET AND SOUR SAUCE

Total yield: 18 servings or 1 ¹/₈ C
Serving size: 1 T
Each serving provides:
Calories: 11
Protein: 0.15 gram
Fat: trace (0.3 gram total/recipe)
Carbohydrate: 2.56 grams

1 C pineapple juice (use reserved juice from canned, juice-packed pineapple)

1 T catsup (low-sodium/low-calorie)

1 T tamari or soy sauce

1 T honey

1 T cornstarch

¹/₄ tsp garlic powder

¹/₄ tsp ground ginger

¹/₄ tsp minced onion flakes

¹/₄ tsp ground turmeric

¹/₈ tsp black pepper

1. In a deep microwave-safe bowl, whisk together pineapple juice, catsup, soy sauce, honey, and cornstarch until dissolved.

2. Add spices and mix well.

3. Microwave on high for 5–7 minutes, stirring frequently as sauce thickens.

Use as a dinner sauce, glaze, or dip for poultry.

◘ MY BEST BARBECUE SAUCE

Total yield: 5 servings or 1 ¹/₄ C
Serving size: ¹/₄ C
Each serving provides:
Calories: 44
Protein: 1.7 grams
Fat: trace (0.5 gram total/recipe)
Carbohydrate: 9.07 grams

1 C tomato sauce (no salt)

¹/₄ C onion, minced

2 medium cloves garlic, minced

2 T nonfat milk

2 T Worcestershire sauce

1 T red wine vinegar

1 T dry cooking sherry

1 T brown sugar substitute

1 tsp dry mustard

1 tsp cornstarch

1 tsp chili powder (no salt)

¹/₂ tsp celery seed

pinch black pepper

1. Combine all ingredients in saucepan and stir well.
2. Simmer over medium-low heat for 30 minutes and serve.
3. For best flavor, refrigerate 1–2 days before using.

This is a versatile sauce. Use it in place of commercial barbecue sauce.

✑ PINCH-HITTING PESTO

A great stand-in for an all-time favorite!

Total yield: 12 servings or ³/₄ C
Serving size: 1 T
Each serving provides:
Calories: 32
Protein: 1.97 grams
Fat: 1.8 grams
Carbohydrate: 1.98 grams

³/₄ C fresh basil,
stemmed and chopped

¹/₄ C fresh parsley, chopped

2 T pine nuts

4 tsp minced garlic
(approximately 5 medium cloves)

5 T grated Parmesan cheese

¹/₄ C oil-free creamy Italian dressing

1. In a food processor, combine basil, parsley, pine nuts, and garlic and process well.
2. Add Parmesan cheese; process well.
3. Add creamy Italian dressing and process until thick.

One ounce of regular pesto sauce contains 155 calories and 15 grams fat. One ounce of Pinch-Hitting Pesto contains 63 calories and 3.6 grams fat.

ᏅᎡ TARTAR SAUCE

Total yield: 9 servings or ¹/₂ + C
Serving size: 1 T
Each serving provides:
Calories: 7
Protein: 0.73 gram
Fat: 0
Carbohydrate: 1.02 grams

¹/₂ C plain nonfat yogurt

¹/₂ dill pickle, chopped

2 tsp onion, finely chopped

1 ¹/₂ tsp fresh parsley, minced

1 tsp lemon juice

¹/₂ tsp dried dill

1. In a small bowl, combine all ingredients.
2. Hand mix with wire whisk.
3. Chill before serving.

Serve with broiled or baked fish, fresh shrimp, or prawns.

∂∂ CITRUS SAUCE

Total yield: 16 servings or 1 C
Serving size: 1 T
Each serving provides:
Calories: 10
Protein: 0.09 gram
Fat: trace (0.5 gram total/recipe)
Carbohydrate: 2.34 grams

1 C fresh-squeezed orange juice

1 T cornstarch

1 T granulated fructose

1 tsp grated orange peel

$^1/_8$ tsp ground ginger

$^1/_8$ tsp nutmeg

1. In a small saucepan, whisk together orange juice and cornstarch.
2. Over medium heat, stir until mixture becomes thick and glossy.
3. Add remaining ingredients, stirring until combined.
4. Remove from heat and serve.

Serve over chilled fruit, pancakes, French toast, or your favorite breakfast item.

CRANBERRY "PLUS" SAUCE

Total yield: 48 servings or 3 C
Serving size: 1 T
Each serving provides:
Calories: 8
Protein: 0.059 gram
Fat: trace (1.2 gram total/recipe)
Carbohydrate: 1.88 grams

1 C water

1 bag cranberries, 12 ounces

1 small ripe banana, mashed well

2 T cornstarch mixed with 2 T cold water

1 T juice concentrate
(apple, raspberry, orange, etc.)

1 T granulated fructose

2 tsp brown sugar substitute (optional)

1 tsp cinnamon

1/4 tsp ground ginger

1. In a medium saucepan, bring water to boil and add cranberries; boil 2 minutes or until cranberries have "popped."
2. Add remaining ingredients and boil over medium heat until thick and bubbly, lightly mashing mixture.
3. Reduce heat to lowest setting; cook for 10 minutes, stirring occasionally.
4. Serve immediately or chill for future use.

This sauce adds zip to turkey meals and sandwiches.

⌖ CREAMY SELECT SAUCE

A quick and healthy alternative to whipped toppings.

Total yield: 9 servings or approximately 1 1/2 C
Serving size: 1 T
Each serving provides:
Calories: 10
Protein: 0.7 gram
Fat: 0
Carbohydrate: 1.8 grams

1/2 C plain nonfat yogurt

1 tsp powdered nonfat milk

2 packages sweetener
(or 1 1/2 tsp granulated fructose)

1 T of your favorite fruit juice concentrate
(apple, raspberry, pineapple, orange, etc.)

1. In a small mixing bowl, combine all ingredients.

2. Whisk together with a wire whisk.

3. Chill and serve.

4. Chill between uses.

ᏧᎦ NATURAL FRUIT TOPPING

Total yield: 7 servings or 1 ³/₄ C
Serving size: ¹/₄ C
Each serving provides:
Calories: 42
Protein: 0.47 gram
Fat: trace (0.5 gram total/recipe)
Carbohydrate: 9.87 grams

1 C orange juice

1 T cornstarch

1 C fresh or water-packed
peaches, chopped

2 tsp granulated fructose

2 T raisins, minced

¹/₄ tsp cinnamon

¹/₄ C crushed pineapple

1. In a medium saucepan, whisk together orange juice and cornstarch.

2. Over medium heat, bring mixture to boil, stirring constantly to avoid burning.

3. When sauce begins to thicken, add peaches, fructose, raisins, and cinnamon.

4. Stir to combine, then remove from heat.

5. Pour mixture into a blender; blend briefly (5 seconds).

6. Pour into bowl and stir in crushed pineapple.

7. Serve this topping either hot or cold.

8. Store in refrigerator.

Try over pancakes, French toast, or as a dessert topping.

✑ WARM VANILLA SAUCE

An elegant touch on fresh chilled fruit or any dessert.

Total yield: 12 servings or ³/₄ C
Serving size: 1 T
Each serving provides:
Calories: 11
Protein: 0.5 gram
Fat: trace (0.4 gram total/recipe)
Carbohydrate: 2.18 grams

³/₄ C nonfat milk

4 tsp granulated fructose

2 ¹/₂ tsp cornstarch

¹/₂ tsp dry Butter Buds

¹/₂ tsp vanilla extract

1. In a deep microwave-safe dish or mug, combine ¹/₂ C milk (reserve ¹/₄ C) and fructose.

2. Microwave 3 minutes on medium setting, stirring *once* during cooking.

3. Whisk together cornstarch and remaining milk; add to sauce.

4. Microwave 2 more minutes on medium setting, stirring *once* during cooking.

5. Remove from microwave; stir in remaining ingredients.

6. Serve warm or chilled.

This sauce cannot be reheated after it has been chilled.

⊙ BLACK BEAN SPREAD

Total yield: 18 servings or 1 1/4 C
Serving size: 1 T
Each serving provides:
Calories: 14
Protein: 1.25 grams
Fat: trace (2 grams total/recipe)
Carbohydrate: 2 grams

1 C cooked black beans, drained

1/3 C plain nonfat yogurt

2 T red onion, minced

2 T green chilies, chopped

1 tsp chili seasoning (no salt)

1 tsp dried minced onion

1/4 tsp garlic powder

1. Mash black beans.
2. Combine all ingredients in a small mixing bowl.
3. Using an electric mixer, blend until smooth.

Use as a spread for pita bread or sandwiches, or as a
vegetable dip for party trays.

❧ CINNAMON SPREAD

Total yield: 12 servings or $^3/_4$ C
Serving size: 1 T
Each serving provides:
Calories: 12
Protein: 1.22 grams
Fat: trace (1.4 grams total/recipe)
Carbohydrate: 1.52 grams

$^1/_2$ C 1 percent cottage cheese

$^1/_4$ C natural applesauce

1 T nonfat milk

1 $^1/_2$ tsp granulated fructose

$^1/_2$ tsp cinnamon

1. Combine all ingredients in a blender; blend until smooth.
2. Chill before serving.

Spread on French toast, pancakes, or your favorite toasted bread.
It also makes a delicious cold fruit dip.

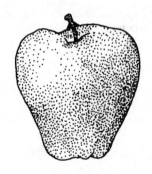

CREAM CHEESE STAND-IN

Total yield: 9 servings or approximately ¹/₂ C
Serving size: 1 T
Each serving provides:
Calories: 17
Protein: 2 grams
Fat: trace (1 gram total/recipe)
Carbohydrate: 2 grams

¹/₂ C 1 percent cottage cheese

3 T nonfat dry milk

2–3 tsp dry Butter Buds (to taste)

1. In small mixing bowl, combine all ingredients.

2. Whip with electric mixer until smooth (2 minutes).

3. Chill before serving.

Spread on bagels and English muffins in place of cream cheese, ricotta cheese, or butter. Add your favorite fresh herb to create your own flavored spread.

ℛ MOCK MAYO

Total yield: 32 servings or 2 C
Serving size: 1 T
Each serving provides:
Calories: 10
Protein: 1.4 grams
Fat: trace (3 grams total/recipe)
Carbohydrate: 0.89 gram

1 1/2 C 1 percent cottage cheese

1/2 C nonfat milk

1 T white wine vinegar

1 tsp prepared mustard (to taste)

1 tsp lemon juice

1. Combine all ingredients in blender; blend until smooth.
2. Chill at least one hour before serving.

Use on sandwiches or mix with tuna for a tangy mayonnaise substitute.

⎌ SOUR CREAM REPLACER

Total yield: 24 servings or 1 1/2 C
Serving size: 1 T
Each serving provides:
Calories: 9
Protein: 1.28 grams
Fat: trace (2 grams total/recipe)
Carbohydrate: 0.78 gram

$^1/_3$ C nonfat milk

1 C 1 percent cottage cheese

1 T lemon juice concentrate

1. Combine all ingredients in blender; blend until smooth.

Use on baked potatoes, sandwiches, or in prepared salads, such as tuna or chicken.

Chapter 2

BREAKFASTS AND BRUNCHES

Breakfasts and Brunches

Berry Interesting
Hot Citrus Ambrosia
Morning Berries!
Spicy Fruit Kabobs
New Potato Hash Browns
Turkey Sausage
Breakfast Pudding
Country Breakfast Rice
Linda's Meal-in-Itself Rice Pudding
Next Day Porridge
Sunday Morning Cereal
Incredible Crepes
Chicken-n-Broccoli Crepes
Creamy Berry Filling
"Bonus" Toast
French Toast
Buttermilk Pancakes
Fast & Famous Potato Pancakes
Hearty Oat Pancakes

⚛ BERRY INTERESTING

A breakfast starter to warm up those taste buds!

Total yield: 4 servings or 2 ²/₃ C
Serving size: ²/₃ C
Each serving provides:
Calories: 100
Protein: 2.19 grams
Fat: 0.3 grams
Carbohydrate: 22.14 grams

1 C blueberries

2 medium red apples, sliced,
cored, and cut into ¹/₂-inch cubes

¹/₂ C seedless green grapes

¹/₂ C Creamy Select Sauce
(p. 22), using raspberry
or apple juice concentrate

1. Toss fruit together in a bowl.

2. Divide fruit evenly into 4 smaller bowls; chill.

3. Prepare Creamy Select Sauce.

4. Pour 2 T Creamy Select Sauce over each dish of fruit and serve.

✆ HOT CITRUS AMBROSIA

Total yield: 4 servings or 3 C
Serving size: $^3/_4$ *C*
Each serving provides:
Calories: 109
Protein: 1.27 grams
Fat: 0.5 gram
Carbohydrate: 24.86 grams

1 $^1/_2$ C blueberries

1 large banana
cut into small tidbits

1 C sliced strawberries

1 C Citrus Sauce (p. 20)

1. Place fruit in a bowl and toss.

2. Divide into four serving dishes and chill.

3. Prepare Citrus Sauce.

4. Before serving, pour $^1/_4$ C hot Citrus Sauce over each dish of fruit.

Serve with hot Country Scones (p. 61).

⊘ MORNING BERRIES!

A refreshing idea.

Total yield: 2 servings or 2 C
Serving size: 1 C
Each serving provides:
Calories: 45
Protein: 0.9 gram
Fat: 0.2 gram
Carbohydrate: 9.9 grams

2 C fresh strawberries, hulled

5 sprigs fresh mint leaves

1. In a small saucepan, boil a small amount of water.
2. Place berries and mint in a steamer basket, place basket in the saucepan, and steam for 6 minutes.
3. Transfer steamed berries to serving bowls.
4. Serve warm.

Great with Homecoming Cinnamon Bread (p. 80).

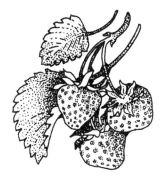

❧ SPICY FRUIT KABOBS

A sensational brunch booster!

Total yield: 4 kabobs
Serving size: 1 kabob
Each serving provides:
Calories: 64
Protein: 0.73 gram
Fat: trace (1.5 grams total/recipe)
Carbohydrate: 14.43 grams

8 whole large strawberries

8 chunks pineapple (2 slices)

8 (1-inch) honeydew melon
cubes ($^1/_4$ melon)

1 banana, cut into 8 pieces

2 T diet maple syrup

1 $^1/_2$ T lemon juice

$^1/_4$ tsp ground red pepper

1. Arrange fruit on four skewers, alternating colors.

2. In small bowl, mix syrup, juice, and pepper.

3. Brush kabobs with juice mixture.

4. Broil 5 minutes, 4 to 5 inches from broiler.

5. Remove from broiler; brush fruit again, then broil 2–3 minutes more.

6. Serve hot, reserving extra sauce for dipping.

Other favorite fruits may be used on these kabobs.

๛ NEW POTATO HASH BROWNS

Total yield: 3 servings
Serving size: ¹/₃ skillet contents
Each serving provides:
Calories: 85
Protein: 3 grams
Fat: 0.1 gram
Carbohydrates: 18 grams

2 medium new potatoes,
shredded

1 egg white

2 T onion, minced

1 ¹/₂ tsp lite soy sauce

1 T water

pepper, to taste

1. In a bowl, combine all ingredients and mix well.
2. Heat a nonstick skillet over medium heat.
3. Pour ingredients into pan and cook until underside is brown.
4. Turn potatoes and brown other side.

Serve with low-salt/low-calorie catsup.

ℭ TURKEY SAUSAGE

Total yield: 6 patties
Serving size: 1 (¹/₂-inch-thick) patty
Each serving provides:
Calories: 88
Protein: 15.25 grams
Fat: 3 grams
Carbohydrate: 0

1 pound ground turkey (96 percent fat free)

1 tsp lite soy sauce

¹/₂ tsp crushed sage

¹/₂ tsp dried onion flakes

¹/₂ tsp garlic powder

¹/₄ tsp black pepper

¹/₄ tsp dry mustard (optional)

¹/₄ tsp crushed red pepper flakes

¹/₄ tsp fennel or anise seeds

¹/₈ tsp salt

1. Place turkey in a large mixing bowl.

2. Combine the remaining ingredients; pour evenly over turkey.

3. Knead turkey and spices thoroughly.

4. Form 6 patties, each ¹/₂ inch thick.

5. Broil or barbecue, or cook in nonstick skillet at medium to low heat until patties are cooked through and browned on outside.

6. Serve patties with New Potato Hash Browns (p. 37) or Hearty Oat Pancakes (p. 52).

Turkey Sausage can be used as an excellent meat base in stuffing or spaghetti sauce.

⧉ BREAKFAST PUDDING

A special touch for breakfast or brunch.

Total Yield: 4 servings or 2 C
Serving size: 1/2 C
Each serving provides:
Calories: 168
Protein: 6.47 grams
Fat: 0.4 gram
Carbohydrate: 34.6 grams

1 1/2 C Basic Brown Rice (p. 126)

1 1/4 C nonfat milk (reserve 1/4 C)

1 T granulated fructose

1/3 C dried fruit and raisins, chopped

2 egg whites

1/4 tsp each vanilla extract and cinnamon

1. In medium saucepan, combine rice, 1 C milk, and fructose.

2. Cook over medium to low heat for 20 minutes, stirring occasionally. *Do not scorch milk.*

3. Reduce heat to low and stir in dried fruit.

4. Lightly whisk together reserved 1/4 C milk and egg whites; combine with rice mixture.

5. Cook 2 minutes, stirring constantly. *Do not allow mixture to boil.*

6. Remove from heat and stir in cinnamon and vanilla.

7. Cover and let stand 4–5 minutes; serve warm.

This is a great morning starter or side dish, and a tasty way to use brown rice leftovers.

⚝ COUNTRY BREAKFAST RICE

Total yield: 6 servings or 3 C
Serving size: 1/2 C
Each serving provides:
Calories: 100
Protein: 5.37 grams
Fat: 0.6 gram
Carbohydrate: 18.28 grams

1 1/2 C Basic Brown Rice (p. 126)*

1 medium red apple, cored, cut in 1/2-inch cubes

1/2 C 1 percent cottage cheese

3 egg whites

1 T water

2 tsp cinnamon

1 tsp granulated fructose

1 T apple juice concentrate

1. Preheat oven to 350°F.
2. Spray a 1 1/2-quart casserole with nonstick cooking spray.
3. Combine all ingredients, except apple juice concentrate, in large mixing bowl.
4. Stir by hand, mixing thoroughly.
5. Pour mixture into prepared 1 1/2-quart casserole dish, spreading mix evenly.
6. Bake 30 minutes and remove from oven.
7. Fluff rice with fork; pour apple juice concentrate over rice.
8. Serve warm.

*Save time by preparing rice the night before.

⌒ LINDA'S MEAL-IN-ITSELF RICE PUDDING

Total yield: 4 servings
Serving size: approximately 1 C
Each serving provides:
Calories: 271
Protein: 11.43 grams
Fat: 1.9 grams
Carbohydrate: 52 grams

2 C Basic Brown Rice (p. 126)

¹/₂ C raisins, minced

3 egg whites and 1 egg yolk
(4 whites may be substituted for a less rich pudding)

1–2 tsp granulated fructose (to taste)

2 C nonfat milk

1 tsp vanilla

1. Mix rice and raisins in a saucepan.

2. In a mixing bowl, whip eggs and fructose with wire whisk until frothy (about 1 minute).

3. Add milk and vanilla to egg mixture; combine with rice mixture.

4. Cook over medium heat, stirring constantly with a wooden spoon until pudding begins to coat sides of pan. *Caution—the milk/egg mixture scorches easily.*

5. Gradually reduce heat, still stirring constantly, as pudding thickens and reaches a very gentle boil.

6. Turn off heat, cover pan, and let stand for about 10 minutes. Serve warm.

This hearty, satisfying dish is equally well suited to breakfast, lunch or dinner, especially on a cold winter day.

ᐵ NEXT DAY PORRIDGE

Make your mornings easy with this overnight sensation!

Total yield: 2 servings or 2 C
Serving size: 1 C
Each serving provides:
Calories: 215
Protein: 4.9 grams
Fat: 0.4 gram
Carbohydrate: 47.95 grams

$^1/_4$ C raw cracked bulgur

$^1/_4$ C quick grits

1 T wheat germ

1 T dark molasses

2 T raisins

1 $^1/_2$ C water

The night before:

1. Combine all ingredients in a saucepan.
2. Cover and refrigerate overnight.

The next morning:

1. Bring to boil and reduce heat to low.
2. Allow to cook 12 minutes, stirring constantly.
3. Serve hot.

⬗ SUNDAY MORNING CEREAL

Total yield: 4 bowls
Serving size: approximately 1 C
Each serving provides:
Calories: 226
Protein: 7.78 grams
Fat: 3 grams
Carbohydrate: 41.97 grams

1 medium banana, sliced

1 medium apple, diced

$^1/_2$ tsp grated orange peel

1 $^1/_3$ C rolled oats

$^2/_3$ C oat bran

2 T raisins

2 T golden raisins or dried cherries

1 tsp cinnamon

$^1/_4$ tsp maple flavoring or extract

pinch nutmeg

cinnamon sticks

1. In a deep saucepan, bring 4 C water to boil.

2. Add banana, apple, and orange peel; bring to boil again.

3. Reduce heat to medium to achieve a low boil.

4. Add remaining ingredients, except cinnamon sticks; cook 8 minutes, stirring frequently.

5. Remove from heat; cover and let stand 3–4 minutes.

6. Garnish with cinnamon sticks and serve.

Ꮼ INCREDIBLE CREPES

Total yield: 16–18 crepes
Serving size: 1 crepe
Each serving provides:
Calories: 40
Protein: 2.12 grams
Fat: 0.4 gram
Carbohydrate: 6.98 grams

1 C buckwheat flour

1 $^1/_3$ C nonfat milk

2 egg whites

1 egg yolk

1. Combine ingredients in a bowl; beat with hand beater until blended.
2. Spray 6-inch skillet with nonstick cooking spray; heat skillet, then remove from heat.
3. Spoon 2 T batter into skillet; lift and tilt skillet to spread batter evenly.
4. Return skillet to heat and brown one side of crepe.
5. Invert pan over paper towel to remove crepe.
6. Repeat until batter is gone (spray skillet every third crepe; avoid spraying when pan is hot).
7. Fill with Creamy Berry Filling (p. 47).

Crepes can be frozen. Stack them, alternating each crepe between two layers of waxed paper. Wrap the stack in an air-tight, moisture-proof bag. Place bag in a plastic container and freeze. Crepes will store frozen for 45 days. Thaw 90 minutes at room temperature before using.

∽ CHICKEN-N-BROCCOLI CREPES

Total yield: 4 crepes
Serving size: 1 crepe
Each serving provides:
Calories: 154
Protein: 15.5 grams
Fat: 2.6 grams
Carbohydrate: 17.15 grams

4 Incredible Crepes (p. 44)

Sauce:
2 T diced onion
1 tsp lite soy sauce combined with 1 tsp water
1 ¼ C nonfat milk
1 T cornstarch
pinch paprika
2 T grated Parmesan cheese
1 T dry white wine
2 T sliced mushrooms, fresh or canned

Filling:
1 C Quick Cooked Chicken (p. 142), finely chopped*
1 C steamed broccoli, chopped*

*To save time, prepare and cook chicken and broccoli the night before. Warm in microwave before using.

(continues)

Sauce:

1. Place onions, soy sauce, and water in skillet; cook onions until tender.
2. Combine milk and cornstarch and add to saucepan.
3. Cook until thick and bubbly, stirring often.
4. Add paprika, cheese, and wine, stirring until cheese melts.
5. Remove ¹/₃ C sauce and set aside.
6. Add mushrooms to saucepan and stir.

Filling:

1. Combine chicken, broccoli, and reserved ¹/₃ C sauce.

Assembly:

1. Spread ¹/₂ C filling over unbrowned side of crepe; roll up crepe; place seam side down in skillet; repeat with remaining crepes.
2. Drizzle sauce over crepes, cover skillet, and cook over low heat until bubbly.

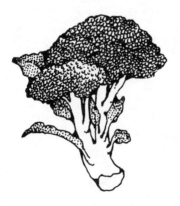

ᥰ CREAMY BERRY FILLING

A great crepe filler!

Total yield: 4 servings
Serving size: 1 crepe
Each serving provides:
Calories: 120
Protein: 8.6 grams
Fat: 1.25 grams
Carbohydrate: 18.59 grams

$^1/_2$ C lowfat ricotta cheese

$^1/_2$ C 1 percent cottage cheese

1 T granulated fructose

$^1/_4$ tsp lemon juice concentrate

$^1/_4$ tsp grated lemon peel (optional)

$^1/_4$ tsp cinnamon

pinch nutmeg

1 $^1/_2$ C fresh strawberries, sliced,
(or your favorite berries)

4 Incredible Crepes (p. 44)

1. In a large mixing bowl, using an electric mixer, whip ricotta and cottage cheese until nearly smooth (2–3 minutes).

2. Add remaining ingredients except berries and crepes; blend for 30 seconds.

3. Gently fold in 1 C berries, and reserve remaining $^1/_2$ C berries to garnish. Reserve $^1/_4$ C filling and set aside.

4. Spoon a line of filling down center of each crepe.

5. Roll crepe around filling; place 1 T of reserved mix on top of each crepe. Garnish with reserved fresh berries and serve.

At 18 calories per tablespoon, this filling may also be used on pancakes or as a chilled fruit topping.

⧉ "BONUS" TOAST

A French toast lover's dream!

Total yield: 4 servings
Serving size: 1 slice
Each serving provides:
Calories: 110
Protein: 6.4 grams
Fat: 0.6 grams
Carbohydrate: 19.8 grams

4 (1 $^1/_2$-inch) slices French bread,
sliced from a baguette

$^1/_4$ C (or 4 T) your favorite natural fruit preserves

4 egg whites

$^1/_2$ C nonfat milk

3 T evaporated skimmed milk

1 tsp cinnamon

$^1/_2$ tsp vanilla extract

1. Cut a 2-inch pocket into the top of the hard crust of each bread slice (do not cut through to other side).

2. Spoon in 1 T natural fruit preserves.

3. Place all slices in pie tin.

4. Whisk remaining ingredients together; pour evenly over bread.

5. Cover and refrigerate 1–2 hours *(for best results, recipe can be made night before, allowing bread to soak overnight)*.

6. Brown slices in nonstick skillet over medium heat, turning once.

7. Serve warm.

ও FRENCH TOAST

Total yield: *4 servings*
Serving size: *1 slice*
Each serving provides:
Calories: *89*
Protein: *5.6 grams*
Fat: *0.7 grams*
Carbohydrate: *15.07 grams*

3 egg whites

2 T nonfat milk

1 T 1.5 percent buttermilk

1 T orange juice concentrate

$^1/_2$ tsp cinnamon

$^1/_4$ tsp vanilla extract

pinch nutmeg

4 slices cracked wheat or whole grain bread
(for best results, allow bread to sit out overnight
before use; dry bread absorbs more liquid)

1. Spray 11-inch skillet with nonstick cooking spray.

2. Whisk together all ingredients except bread.

3. Place 2 bread slices in pie tin and pour half of liquid
   mixture over them.

4. Let stand 4 minutes.

5. Heat skillet over medium heat; place soaked bread in skillet
   and brown on each side.

6. Repeat with remaining bread slices.

7. Serve with Cinnamon Spread (p. 26), Citrus Sauce (p. 20),
   or natural applesauce.

8. Garnish with fresh fruit.

๛ BUTTERMILK PANCAKES

Total yield: 12 servings
Serving size: 1 pancake
Each serving provides:
Calories: 48
Protein: 2.17 grams
Fat: 0.4 gram
Carbohydrate: 8.93 grams

³/₄ C flour

¹/₄ C oat bran

1 tsp baking powder

1 tsp each granulated fructose and baking soda

¹/₈ tsp salt

3 egg whites

1 ¹/₄ C 1 percent buttermilk, if available
(or a mixture of 1.5 percent buttermilk and nonfat milk)

1. In a mixing bowl, combine all dry ingredients.
2. In a small bowl, beat egg whites 1–2 minutes with wire whisk until frothy.
3. Add buttermilk to whites; beat another 2 minutes.
4. Gently stir milk and egg mixture into dry ingredients; stir only until blended. *Do not overmix (batter will be lumpy, but lumps will cook out).*
5. Let batter stand 15 minutes.
6. Spray skillet with nonstick cooking spray; warm skillet over medium to medium-low heat.
7. Pour ¹/₄ C batter into skillet for each pancake; pancakes will cook slowly; let all bubbles rise and cook out before turning over.

Serve with warm applesauce, fresh blueberries, Creamy Select Sauce (p. 22), or your favorite low-calorie syrup.

ᕼ FAST & FAMOUS POTATO PANCAKES

Total yield: 4 servings, 20 pancakes
Serving size: 5 (3-inch) pancakes
Each serving provides:
Calories: 125
Protein: 5 grams
Fat: trace (1 gram total/recipe)
Carbohydrate: 24 grams

3 large egg whites

$^2/_3$ C chopped red onion

2 T + 2 tsp flour

$^1/_2$ tsp salt

$^1/_4$ tsp baking powder

3 C cubed raw potatoes ($^1/_2$-inch cubes)

1. Place egg whites, onion, flour, salt, baking powder, and $^1/_2$ C potatoes in blender.

2. Cover and blend on highest speed until smooth.

3. Add remaining potatoes; cover and blend on pulse or in 4 2-second cycles at medium speed until chunky.

4. After each 2-second cycle, remove lid and push potatoes to bottom of blender.

5. Spray pan or griddle with nonstick cooking spray; heat pan to medium-high heat.

6. Pour one heaping tablespoon batter onto hot surface; cook 4 minutes on each side or until golden brown.

7. Serve with Sour Cream Replacer (p. 29), low-sodium/low-calorie catsup, or your favorite low-calorie syrup.

This batter does not store well. Use immediately.

❧ HEARTY OAT PANCAKES

Total yield: 16 pancakes
Serving size: 1 (4-inch) pancake
Each serving provides:
Calories: 70
Protein: 3.9 grams
Fat: 0.4 grams
Carbohydrate: 12.7 grams

1 C rolled oats
(or 1/2 C oat bran and 1/2 C rolled oats)
1 C oat flour (unbleached flour optional)
1 1/2 tsp cinnamon
1 T granulated fructose
1 1/2 tsp baking soda
1 large banana, very ripe
2 tsp vanilla extract
1 1/2 C plain nonfat yogurt
4 egg whites
2 T dry Butter Buds

1. Spray 9-inch skillet with nonstick cooking spray.

2. Combine oats, oat flour, cinnamon, fructose, and baking soda in large mixing bowl.

3. In small bowl, mash banana with fork; add vanilla and mix well.

4. Combine banana mixture with dry ingredients.

5. Add yogurt and mix to combine.

6. With an electric mixer, whip egg whites until peaks form.

7. Blend ¹/₃ of egg whites into batter until *just* combined. *Do not overmix.*

8. Gently fold in remaining egg whites and Butter Buds.

9. Cook over medium heat, turning only once.

Serve with natural applesauce or your favorite low calorie syrup.

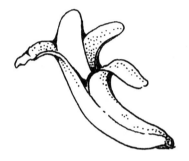

Chapter 3

THE
BREAD
BOX

The Bread Box

ᢒ QUICK BREADS

Banana Bread

Basic Bran Muffins

Bran Bread

Hint-of-Honey Bread

Country Scones

Sunshine Scones

Linda's Applesauce
Oatmeal Bread

Old-Fashioned Cornbread

Tija's Favorite Cornbread

One-Hour Oat Bread

Raisin Wheat Treat

Twisted Apple Muffins

YEAST BREADS ᢒ

Bite-Size Biscuits

Farmer's French

Homecoming
Cinnamon Bread

Onion Bread

Surprise Drop Biscuits

Eight-Grain Raisin Roll

⁊ BANANA BREAD

Total yield: 1 loaf (10 slices)
Serving size: 1 slice
Each serving provides:
Calories: 75
Protein: 4 grams
Fat: 0.35 gram
Carbohydrate: 13.96 grams

$3/4$ C whole wheat flour

$1/3$ C wheat germ

1 T baking powder

$1/2$ tsp each baking soda and cinnamon

pinch salt

3 large egg whites

1 large (or 2 small) very ripe bananas

1 C plain nonfat yogurt

2 T granulated fructose

$1/4$ tsp grated orange peel

1. Preheat oven to 350°F. Spray 8 $1/2$-by-4 $1/2$-by-2-inch (medium) loaf pan with nonstick cooking spray.

2. In a large bowl, combine flour, wheat germ, baking powder, baking soda, cinnamon, and salt.

3. In a blender, combine egg whites, banana, yogurt, fructose, and orange peel and blend until smooth (30–60 seconds).

4. Pour liquid mixture into dry ingredients; beat with electric mixer until smooth (1–2 minutes).

5. Pour batter into prepared pan and bake for 33–36 minutes.

6. Remove bread from oven; allow to cool 5 minutes in pan. Then remove bread from pan; finish cooling on wire rack.

ॐ BASIC BRAN MUFFINS

Total yield: 8 muffins
Serving size: 1 muffin
Each serving provides:
Calories: 107
Protein: 4 grams
Fat: 0.4 gram
Carbohydrate: 21.85 grams

1 C whole wheat flour

$^1/_2$ C unbleached flour

$^1/_2$ C wheat bran

$^1/_2$ tsp baking powder

$^1/_2$ tsp baking soda

$^3/_4$ C nonfat yogurt

$^1/_4$ C water

3 T molasses

1. Preheat oven to 400°F.

2. Spray 8 muffin tin cups with nonstick cooking spray.

3. In a large bowl, combine flours, wheat bran, baking powder, and baking soda.

4. In a small bowl, whisk together yogurt, water, and molasses.

5. Fold liquid mixture into dry ingredients and mix with a few quick strokes until just combined.

6. Fill muffin tins $^3/_4$ full.

7. Bake 15–18 minutes, or until golden brown.

8. Remove from oven and cool 5 minutes on wire rack.

9. Remove muffins from tins and allow to cool thoroughly.

⟆ BRAN BREAD

Total yield: 1 loaf (12 slices)
Serving size: 1 slice
Each serving provides:
Calories: 79
Protein: 3.1 grams
Fat: 0.4 gram
Carbohydrate: 15.75 grams

1 $^1/_4$ C whole wheat flour

$^3/_4$ C wheat bran

$^1/_2$ tsp salt

$^3/_4$ tsp baking soda

2 T brown sugar substitute

3 T molasses

1 C nonfat buttermilk

$^1/_4$ C raisins

1. Preheat oven to 350°F. Spray 6 $^1/_2$-by-4 $^1/_2$-by-2-inch (small) loaf pan with nonstick cooking spray.

2. In a large bowl, combine flour, wheat bran, salt, baking soda, and brown sugar substitute; mix well.

3. In a small bowl, add molasses to buttermilk and mix well.

4. Fold liquid mixture into dry ingredients until just combined. Fold in raisins.

5. Spoon batter into prepared loaf pan and bake for 45–50 minutes.

6. Remove bread from oven and cool in pan on wire rack for 20 minutes. Remove loaf from pan and invert to cool.

This bread is also delicious with $^1/_2$ C apples substituted for the raisins.

ᘒ HINT-OF-HONEY BREAD

Total yield: 2 loaves (32 slices)
Serving size: 1 (¹/₂-inch) slice
Each serving provides:
Calories: 51
Protein: 2.22 grams
Fat: trace (3.5 grams total/recipe or 1.75 grams total/loaf)
Carbohydrate: 10.28 grams

2 C whole wheat flour

1 ¹/₂ C enriched all-purpose flour

1 tsp baking powder

1 tsp baking soda

1 tsp salt

2 C plain nonfat yogurt

1 T honey

2 T caraway seeds

1. Preheat oven to 350°F.

2. Spray two 8 ¹/₂-by-4 ¹/₂-by-2-inch (medium) loaf pans with nonstick cooking spray.

3. In a large bowl, sift together flours, baking powder, baking soda, and salt.

4. Add yogurt, honey, and caraway seeds to dry ingredients.

5. Mix well with fork; dough will be sticky.

6. Divide dough in two and place halves in prepared loaf pans.

7. Bake for 65–75 minutes.

8. Remove from oven and cool on wire rack.

This natural bread has a simple yet wholesome flavor. If caraway seeds aren't your favorite, omit or substitute other seeds.

ℭ COUNTRY SCONES

Total yield: 8 scones
Serving size: 1 scone
Each serving provides:
Calories: 145
Protein: 7 grams
Fat: 0.7 gram
Carbohydrate: 27.68 grams

1 $^1/_2$ C unbleached flour

$^1/_3$ C rolled oats

2 T cornstarch

2 T granulated fructose

1 tsp baking soda

$^3/_4$ tsp cinnamon

$^1/_2$ tsp grated orange peel

2 crushed cardamom seeds

2 pinches salt

$^3/_4$ C 1 percent cottage cheese

3 large egg whites

3 T plain nonfat yogurt

$^1/_4$ C raisins, minced

1. Preheat oven to 425°F.

2. Lightly dust a baking sheet with flour.

3. In a large bowl, combine flour, oats, cornstarch, fructose, baking soda, cinnamon, orange peel, cardamon, and salt; mix well.

4. Cut in cottage cheese until mixture is crumbly.

5. In a small bowl, whisk together egg whites, yogurt, and raisins.

(continues)

6. Add wet mixture to dry mixture; combine with a fork to form a sticky dough.

7. Turn dough onto floured baking sheet; lightly dust top of dough with flour and pat dough into an 8- to 9-inch circle, $1/2$ inch thick.

8. Using a sharp knife, score or slice the circle into 8 pie wedges. *Do not separate wedges.*

9. Bake 14 minutes, then remove and cover scone round with aluminum foil.

10. Return to oven; bake an additional 4–6 minutes.

11. Remove from oven and allow to cool 10 minutes on a wire rack before cutting.

12. To serve, cut scones along pre-scored lines.

For optimum freshness, slice scones as needed from round.

◈ SUNSHINE SCONES

Total yield: 8 scones
Serving size: 1 scone
Each serving provides:
Calories: 155
Protein: 8 grams
Fat: 0.8 gram
Carbohydrate: 28.95 grams

1 ³/₄ C unbleached flour

3 T cornstarch

1 tsp baking soda

¹/₄ tsp nutmeg

³/₄ C 1 percent cottage cheese

¹/₂ C lowfat peach yogurt,
fruit juice sweetened

¹/₄ C golden raisins, minced

3 large egg whites

1 ¹/₂ tsp granulated fructose

¹/₈ tsp nutmeg

1. Preheat oven to 425°F.
2. Lightly dust a nonstick baking sheet with flour.
3. In a large bowl, combine flour, cornstarch, baking soda, and nutmeg; mix well.
4. Cut in cottage cheese until mixture is crumbly.
5. In a small bowl, whisk together yogurt, raisins, and egg whites.
6. Add wet mixture to dry mixture; combine with a fork to form a sticky dough.

(continues)

7. Turn dough onto floured baking sheet; lightly dust top of dough with flour and pat dough into a 9-inch circle, $^3/_4$ inch thick.

8. Combine fructose and nutmeg, sprinkle over top of dough.

9. Using a large knife, score or slice circle into 8 pie wedges. *Do not separate wedges.*

10. Bake 13–14 minutes; remove and cover scone round with aluminum foil.

11. Return scones to oven and bake 4–6 minutes.

12. Remove from oven and allow to cool 10 minutes on wire rack before cutting.

13. To serve, cut scones along pre-existing scored lines.

For optimum freshness, slice scones as needed from round.

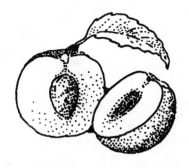

LINDA'S APPLESAUCE OATMEAL BREAD

Total yield: 1 loaf (18 slices)
Serving size: 1 (¹/₂-inch) slice
Each serving provides:
Calories: 103
Protein: 3.3 grams
Fat: 2.1 grams
Carbohydrate: 17.72 grams

¹/₃ C raisins

³/₄ C white flour

¹/₄ C soy flour

4 tsp baking powder

¹/₄ tsp baking soda

1 C whole wheat flour

1 C rolled oats

1 to 1 ¹/₄ tsp total spices:
either all cinnamon or any combination of
cinnamon, nutmeg, cloves, cardamom, and ginger

2 egg whites

2 T oil

³/₄ C natural applesauce

¹/₄ C honey

³/₄ C water

1. Preheat oven to 350°F.

2. Spray 9-by-5-by-3-inch loaf pan with nonstick cooking spray.

(continues)

3. In a small bowl, cover raisins with hot water and allow to soak for 10–15 minutes.

4. In a large bowl, sift together white flour, soy flour, baking powder, and baking soda; sift again.

5. Add whole wheat flour, rolled oats, and spices of your choice to sifted flours; mix well.

6. In medium bowl, combine egg whites, oil, applesauce, honey, and water; beat well.

7. Drain raisins and add to liquid mixture.

8. Combine wet mixture with flour mixture; stir just until moistened.

9. Pour batter into prepared loaf pan.

10. Bake for 50–60 minutes or until a toothpick inserted in center comes out clean.

11. Cool in pan for 15 minutes, then turn out on wire rack to cool thoroughly before slicing.

12. Store in a cool place.

∽ OLD-FASHIONED CORNBREAD

Total yield: 15 pieces
Serving size: 1 piece
Each serving provides:
Calories: 83
Protein: 3.1 grams
Fat: 0.6 gram
Carbohydrate: 16.3 grams

1 C ground yellow cornmeal

1 C unbleached flour

2 T granulated fructose

1 T baking powder

$^1/_4$ tsp baking soda

pinch salt

3 egg whites

$^1/_2$ C 1 $^1/_2$ percent buttermilk

$^1/_2$ C + 2 T nonfat milk

1 C canned or thawed frozen corn

1. Preheat oven to 400° F. Spray 13-by-9-by-2-inch pan with nonstick cooking spray.

2. In a large bowl, combine cornmeal, flour, fructose, baking powder, baking soda, and salt and mix thoroughly.

3. In a small bowl, whisk egg whites for 1 minute. Add both milks to egg whites and whisk to combine.

4. Add liquid mixture to dry mixture; stir by hand until *just* combined; add corn and stir. Pour into prepared pan and spread evenly.

6. Bake 25 minutes and remove; cool 15 minutes on wire rack. before slicing. Serve warm; cornbread hardens as it cools.

Great with chili and stews (see Soups and Stews section, p. 99).

℞ TIJA'S FAVORITE CORNBREAD

A fluffy, light cornbread.

Total yield: 15 pieces
Serving size: 1 piece
Each serving provides:
Calories: 94
Protein: 4.9 grams
Fat: 0.6 gram
Carbohydrate: 17.25 grams

5 egg whites

1 C 1 percent cottage cheese

1 C "light style" creamed corn
(80 calories per $^1/_2$ cup)

1 C ground yellow cornmeal

1 C unbleached flour

2 $^1/_2$ T granulated fructose

1 T baking powder

pinch salt

$^1/_2$ C frozen corn, thawed

1. Preheat oven to 375°F. Spray a 13-by-9-by-2-inch pan with nonstick cooking spray.

2. With an electric mixer, blend egg whites and cottage cheese until smooth; stir in creamed corn by hand.

3. In a large bowl, combine remaining ingredients, except frozen corn, and mix thoroughly.

4. Add wet ingredients to dry ingredients, stirring by hand until *just* combined. Stir in corn.

5. Pour batter into prepared pan and spread evenly. Bake for 25 minutes.

Ꮺ ONE-HOUR OAT BREAD

An easy soda bread.

Total yield: 1 loaf (15 slices)
Serving size: 1 slice
Each serving provides:
Calories: 77
Protein: 3.46 grams
Fat: 0.6 gram
Carbohydrate: 14.44 grams

1 $1/4$ C unbleached flour
(reserve 2 T for kneading)

1 tsp salt

1 tsp baking soda

$1/2$ tsp baking powder

1 C oat flour

$1/2$ C rolled oats

1 C 1 $1/2$ percent buttermilk

2 egg whites

1. Preheat oven to 350°F.

2. Spray baking sheet with nonstick cooking spray.

3. In a large mixing bowl, sift flour, salt, baking soda, and baking powder.

4. Add oat flour and oats; mix well.

5. In a small bowl, combine buttermilk and eggs and whisk lightly.

6. Add liquid mixture to dry mixture, combining with a fork to form a sticky dough.

7. Lightly flour a bread board using one of the reserved tablespoons of flour.

(continues)

8. Turn out dough and knead one minute *(dough will remain sticky)*, using the last reserved tablespoon of flour, if needed.

9. Roll into ball and place on prepared baking sheet.

10. Sprinkle top with a few oats and lightly dust with flour.

11. Bake 30–32 minutes or until browned.

12. Remove from oven and cool on wire rack.

ᏧᎳ RAISIN WHEAT TREAT

A wholesome bread with a natural fruit taste.

Yield: 2 loaves (20 slices)
Serving size: 1 (³/₄-inch) slice
Each serving provides:
Calories: 78
Protein: 2.51 grams
Fat: 0.3 gram (3 grams total/loaf)
Carbohydrate: 16.65 grams

1 ¹/₂ C whole wheat flour

¹/₄ C unbleached flour

¹/₃ C oat bran

¹/₄ C wheat germ

2 tsp baking powder

1 tsp baking soda

2 tsp cinnamon

2 tsp granulated fructose

3 egg whites

³/₄ C evaporated skimmed milk

¹/₃ C orange juice concentrate

1 T molasses

¹/₄ C raisins, chopped

1 granny smith apple, peeled,
cored, and finely chopped

1. Preheat oven to 350°F.

2. Spray two 8 ¹/₂-by-4 ¹/₂-by-2-inch (medium) loaf pans with
   nonstick cooking spray.

(continues)

3. In a large bowl, combine flours, oat bran, wheat germ, baking powder, baking soda, cinnamon, and fructose.

4. In a small bowl, combine egg whites, milk, orange juice concentrate, and molasses; beat for 1 minute with electric mixer.

5. Combine wet mixture with dry ingredients and blend well with electric mixer.

6. With a wooden spoon, stir in raisins and apple bits.

7. Divide dough evenly into two prepared loaf pans.

8. Bake for 30–35 minutes, or until toothpick inserted in center comes out clean.

9. Remove from pans and cool on wire rack.

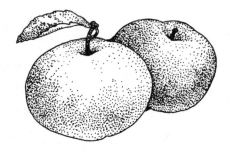

☙ TWISTED APPLE MUFFINS

Total yield: 10 muffins
Serving size: 1 muffin
Each serving provides:
Calories: 120
Protein: 4.4 grams
Fat: 0.8 gram
Carbohydrate: 23.8 grams

Muffins:

1 C rolled oats

$^1/_2$ C whole wheat flour

$^1/_2$ C all-purpose unbleached flour

1 T soy flour

$^1/_4$ C wheat germ

2 rounded T granulated fructose

1 T baking powder

2 tsp cinnamon

1 C unsweetened crushed pineapple, drained

$^1/_2$ C natural applesauce

1 large egg white

$^3/_4$ C nonfat milk

Topping:

1 heaping T rolled oats

honey

1. Preheat oven to 400°F.
2. Spray 10 muffin tin cups with nonstick cooking spray.

(continues)

3. In a large bowl, combine oats, flours, wheat germ, fructose, baking powder, and cinnamon.

4. In a small bowl, combine pineapple and applesauce.

5. Fold wet ingredients into dry ingredients and mix *just* until moistened.

6. In a small bowl, whip egg white and nonfat milk by hand.

7. Add to batter and stir *just* until combined.*

8. Fill muffin tins ³/₄ C full.

9. *For topping:* Before baking, drop ¹/₄ C tsp honey over each muffin and sprinkle a few oats on top.

10. Bake for 25 minutes or until golden brown.

11. Remove from oven and cool 5 minutes on wire rack.

12. Remove muffins from tins and allow to cool thoroughly. before storing.

13. Store in airtight plastic containers in a cool place.

When combining moist and dry ingredients, always stir until just combined. Overmixing may result in tough muffins.

YEAST BREADS ∂ᴼ ∂ᴼ ∂ᴼ ∂ᴼ ∂ᴼ

If you're a first-time yeast user, the information below will prove invaluable to your success with the recipes that follow.

Active dry yeast is sold in two forms, regular and rapid rise. Both are used in the yeast breads in the following section.

To activate:
> Yeast is either sprinkled over and dissolved in 105° to 115°F water, or sprinkled into dry ingredients and activated by adding 120° to 130°F liquid to the dry mixture. A cooking thermometer and glass measuring cup are the best assurance of a correct water temperature. Boil water, pour it into a measuring cup, and allow to cool to the appropriate temperature for each recipe.

> *Caution:* Yeast is extremely temperamental and delicate! Your recipe's success will depend upon how diligently you follow recipe instructions. Correct water temperature and a warm environment are a must—and worth the extra time in compliments! If the water you use to activate the yeast is too hot, it will destroy the yeast. However, cold water will not properly activate yeast. Finally, prepare bread in a warm environment. A draft can ruin dough.

Kneading:
> Adding reserved flour during the kneading process is the only way to measure how much flour actually is used. (All flours vary in moisture content.) Spray your fingertips lightly with nonstick cooking spray to prevent sticking, or lightly flour your hands. Follow the recipe's required kneading time. Overkneading will result in coarse bread. Knead moderately by folding dough toward you, then pressing it away gently. Repeat this motion for the amount of time specified. Dough should become smooth and elastic.

To rise:
> To ensure a warm "rising" environment quickly, turn your oven on and adjust it to its lowest setting for 90 seconds, then turn it off. Wait two minutes. Cover dough lightly with a cloth

and place it in the oven for the recipe's specified rising time. Be sure to remove bread from the oven *before* preheating it to bake.

Punching dough:

Some recipes call for punching. When dough has doubled in size, ball your hand and punch once, pushing your hand to the bottom of the dough. The edges will turn to the center and the bottom of the dough will move upward. At this point, follow your recipe. Dough may require a second, brief kneading and another rise period, or the recipe may call for shaping the dough into small pieces and allowing a short rest.

Cooling:

When bread is done baking, remove it from the pan or sheet and allow it to cool on a wire rack. Allow to cool *completely* before storing. To avoid shrinkage, keep breads away from drafts.

Storage:

Let bread cool *completely* before wrapping and storing. Warm bread will draw condensation and molding will start immediately. Breads can be wrapped in plastic and stored in tins with small breathing airholes and kept in a cool place such as a bread box. Both excessive warmth and refrigeration will encourage mold growth on bread. *Note: Since bread recipes in this book do not call for added fats, your breads will have a shorter storage life (5 to 7 days).*

Freezing:

If you choose to freeze your cooked bread, allow it to cool 4 hours before wrapping it tightly in plastic and again in foil. To use, thaw only the amount needed, as breads dry out rapidly after thawing. Allow to thaw at room temperature for 2 hours. Bread may be placed in a warm oven, 275°F for 20 minutes, before serving.

⬟ BITE-SIZE BISCUITS

The great soup mate!

Total yield: 24 (bite-size) biscuits or 12 (average) biscuits
Serving size: 2 (bite-size) biscuits or 1 (average) biscuit
Each serving provides:
Calories: 48
Protein: 1.85 grams
Fat: trace (1.3 grams total/recipe)
Carbohydrate: 10.03 grams

1 1/4 C all-purpose flour

2 tsp dry rapid rise yeast

1 1/2 tsp granulated fructose

1/2 rounded tsp salt

1/2 C nonfat milk

1/4 C water

1. In a small bowl, combine 1 C flour (reserve 1/4 C), yeast, fructose, and salt.

2. In a small saucepan, combine milk and water; heat to 120° to 130°F. *Do not boil.*

3. Add liquid to flour mixture; combine with a fork.

4. Slowly stir in reserved 1/4 C flour by spoonfuls.

5. Using a fork, knead dough in bowl 2 minutes; dough will be sticky.

6. Using a small spoon, drop by rounded spoonfuls onto a nonstick baking sheet.

7. Cover with cloth; let rise 20 minutes in a warm area.

8. Preheat oven to 300°F.

9. Bake 25–30 minutes, or until tops brown. Cool on wire rack.

ॐ FARMER'S FRENCH

A hearty whole-wheat alternative with only a trace of fat.

Total yield: 3 (8-inch) loaves (16 slices/loaf)
Serving size: 1 (¹/₂-inch) slice
Each serving provides:
Calories: 48
Protein: 2.17 grams
Fat: trace (1.8 grams total/loaf)
Carbohydrate: 9.76 grams

1 package dry active yeast

¹/₂ C 115°F (warm) water

1 ¹/₂ C hot water

2 tsp salt

1 C plain nonfat yogurt,
at room temperature

5–6 C whole wheat flour

1. Dissolve yeast in 115°F warm water and let stand 3 minutes.

2. In a large bowl, combine 1 ¹/₂ C hot water and salt.

3. Add yogurt to bowl, stirring well to combine *(mixture should be warm)*.

4. Add dissolved yeast to yogurt mixture.

5. Slowly add 5 C flour and combine with fork *(dough should not be sticky)*.

6. Turn out on floured board and knead for 10 minutes; use remaining cup of flour as needed.

7. Turn dough into a large bowl sprayed with nonstick cooking spray and cover with damp cloth.

8. Let rise for 1 $1/2$ hours in warm area until doubled in size *(Tip: The oven turned on low for 90 seconds, then turned off, works well to create a warm area.)*

9. When doubled in size, punch dough down and remove from bowl.

10. Gently knead dough for about 10 seconds.

11. Form into 3 loaves.

12. Spray 2 nonstick baking sheets with nonstick cooking spray.

13. Lightly sprinkle nonstick baking sheets with oat bran and place loaves on sheet.

14. Cover loaves and let rise for 30 minutes in a warm area.

15. Preheat oven to 365°F.

16. With a sharp knife, cut diagonal slits in tops of loaves every 2 inches.

17. Spray loaves lightly with warm water and bake for 35–45 minutes.

18. Remove from oven and cool loaves on wire rack.

This bread takes an extra long time to rise since it's made with whole-wheat flour. It's worth the wait!

⟨℞ HOMECOMING CINNAMON BREAD

My famous disappearing sensation!

Total yield: 1 (12-inch) loaf (24 slices)
Serving size: 1 (¹/₂-inch) slice
Each serving provides:
Calories: 60
Protein: 1.7 grams
Fat: trace (3 grams total/loaf)
Carbohydrate: 13.02 grams

Dough:

3 C unbleached flour (reserve ¹/₂ C)

1 package rapid rise yeast

2 T dry Butter Buds

2 T granulated fructose

1 tsp salt

1 C 130°F water

1 egg white, at room temperature

Baste:

1 T apple juice concentrate,
at room temperature

Filling:

¹/₂ C raisins

2 tsp cinnamon

1. Spray baking sheet with nonstick cooking spray.

2. In a large glass or ceramic bowl, combine 2 1/2 C unbleached flour, yeast, Butter Buds, fructose, and salt.

3. Add 130°F water and egg white; mix together with a fork.

4. Knead 3–4 minutes in bowl, using reserved 1/2 C flour as needed *(dough should not stick to bowl)*.

5. Lightly flour board and roll out dough into 1/4-inch-thick rectangle (14 by 10 inches).

6. Brush room temperature apple juice over dough.

7. Dot dough with raisins; sprinkle cinnamon evenly over dough.

8. Starting with one of dough's long sides, roll up dough jelly-roll style; completely enclose filling.

9. Place long cylindrical loaf onto prepared baking sheet, pinch ends closed.

10. Using sharp scissors, cut 1-inch diagonal slits into alternate sides of bread, Christmas tree–style.

11. Cover bread with cloth.

12. Let rise 30 minutes in warm area *(oven turned on low for 90 seconds, then turned off, works well to create a warm area)*.

13. Remove from oven and allow to rise 5 minutes more while oven is preheating.

14. Preheat oven to 375°F.

15. Remove cloth and bake bread for 15–18 minutes, or until golden brown.

16. Cool on wire rack.

♋ ONION BREAD

A great snack or a delicious complement to any meal.

Yield: 1 loaf (10 slices)
Serving size: 1 (¹/₄-inch) slice
Each serving provides:
Calories: 114
Protein: 6.43
Fat: 0.4 gram (4 grams total/loaf)
Carbohydrate: 21.17 grams

1 package rapid rise yeast

¹/₄ C warm water (115°F)

1 C 1 percent cottage cheese,
at room temperature

¹/₄ C grated white onion,
at room temperature

1 T fructose

1 ¹/₄ tsp salt

2 egg whites,
at room temperature

2 C + 2 T unsifted flour

1. Spray a 1 ¹/₂-quart glass or ceramic
   casserole dish with nonstick cooking spray.

2. In a small glass dish, dissolve yeast by sprinkling over
   115°F water; let stand for 5 minutes, then gently stir.

3. In a large mixing bowl, blend yeast with remaining
   ingredients, except flour.

4. Form into dough by adding flour slowly, ¹/₂ C at a time,
   mixing with a wooden spoon after each addition.
   Note: Dough may only need 2 cups of flour.

5. Cover dough with cloth.

6. Let rise in a warm area for 30 minutes until doubled in size.

7. Using stirring motion, lightly stir dough down with wooden spoon, forming into a ball.

8. Turn ball into prepared casserole dish.

9. Let rise 15 minutes or until almost doubled in size.

10. Preheat oven to 350°F.

11. Bake for 40–45 minutes or until golden brown.

12. Remove from pan and cool on wire rack.

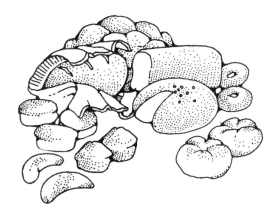

⨍ SURPRISE DROP BISCUITS

Total yield: 15 biscuits
Serving size: 1 biscuit
Each serving provides:
Calories: 87
Protein: 2.87 grams
Fat: 0.2 gram
Carbohydrate: 18.43 grams

2 $^3/_4$ to 3 C all-purpose flour

1 package rapid rise yeast

2 tsp granulated fructose

$^1/_4$ rounded tsp salt

1 C 130°F water

1 egg white, at room temperature

1 small juice orange, peeled, at room temperature

1 tsp grated orange peel

1. In a large bowl, combine 1 C flour (reserve 2 C), yeast, fructose, and salt.

2. Place orange in another bowl; with a knife, slice orange to reduce it to pulp and juice.

3. Add water, egg white, orange, and grated orange peel to flour mixture; stir to combine. Using a fork, gradually stir in remaining flour.

4. Knead by hand for 2 minutes *(dough should be sticky)*.

5. Using a large soup spoon, drop dough by spoonfuls (15) onto a nonstick baking sheet. Cover with cloth and let rise in a warm area for 20 minutes.

6. Preheat oven to 425°F.

7. Bake 8–10 minutes.

8. Remove and cool on wire rack.

ॐ EIGHT-GRAIN RAISIN ROLL

A wonderful change of pace for breakfast!

Total yield: 8 large rolls
Serving size: 1 roll
Each serving provides:
Calories: 160
Protein: 8.23 grams
Fat: 0.5 gram
Carbohydrate: 30.65 grams

1 package rapid rise yeast

$1/4$ C warm water (115°F)

1 C 1 percent cottage cheese, at room temperature

2 large egg whites, at room temperature

$1/3$ C raisins, diced

2 T eight-grain cereal, raw

1 T granulated fructose

1 tsp cinnamon

pinch salt

2 C unsifted, unbleached flour

1. Dissolve yeast by sprinkling it over water; let stand 4–5 minutes, then stir gently.

2. In a large bowl, add all remaining ingredients, except flour; blend slowly to combine.

3. Add flour $1/2$ C at a time, mixing by hand, until dough forms. Knead 3–4 minutes; shape into 8 rolls.

4. Place on nonstick baking sheet; cover and let rise in a warm area 30–40 minutes.

5. Preheat oven to 350°F.

6. Bake 22–25 minutes; cool on wire rack.

Chapter 4

WHO MADE THE SALAD?

Who Made the Salad?

Avant-Garde Albacore
Chicken Salad
Cold Potato Salad
Fancy Fruit Salad
Hot Pasta Salad
Hurry Curry Salad
Seattle Salad
Shrimp-Atizer Salad
"Sweet-Hots" Salad

Ꮞ AVANT-GARDE ALBACORE

Total yield: 2 servings or 1 1/2 C
Serving size: 3/4 C
Each serving provides:
Calories: 130
Protein: 20 grams
Fat: 2 grams
Carbohydrate: 8 grams

1 (6.5-ounce) can albacore tuna,
water-packed, drained

3 T plain nonfat yogurt

1 T prepared mustard

1 T apple juice concentrate

1/2 C celery, diced

1/2 C red bell pepper, diced

1/4 tsp paprika

2 pinches ground cumin

1. In a small bowl, combine all ingredients.

2. Mix well with a fork.

3. Chill.

Serve on lettuce leaves as a side salad, or use as a
sandwich spread.

ᘉ CHICKEN SALAD

Total yield: 2 servings or 2 2/3 C
Serving size: 1 1/3 C
Each serving provides:
Calories: 210
Protein: 31.2 grams
Fat: 3.3 grams
Carbohydrate: 13.88 grams

1 C Quick Cooked Chicken (p. 142), cut into pieces
(approximately 1 breast)

1/3 C red bell pepper, diced

1/3 C celery, diced

20 slices water chestnuts

2 T red onion, chopped

2 T raisins

1/3 C Mock Mayo (p. 28)

pinch of paprika for garnish

1. Toss all ingredients in a mixing bowl.
2. Divide into two portions and chill.
3. Serve on lettuce leaves; garnish with paprika.

Makes a great sandwich spread, too.

❧ COLD POTATO SALAD

An ideal salad for picnics and barbeques.

Total yield: 8 servings or 8 C
Serving size: 1 C
Each serving provides:
Calories: 118
Protein: 2.22 grams
Fat: 0.1 gram
Carbohydrate: 25.03 grams

2 pounds baby new potatoes (7 C)

1 $^{1}/_{4}$ C natural salsa (sugar- and oil-free)
or South Border Salsa (p. 10)

$^{1}/_{2}$ C apple, diced

$^{1}/_{2}$ C jicama root, diced

$^{1}/_{2}$ C pineapple tidbits

$^{1}/_{3}$ C fresh cilantro,
chopped

2 T red onion, diced

1 T chili pepper, diced

1 tsp ground cumin

$^{1}/_{2}$ tsp ground ginger

1. Cut potatoes into $^{1}/_{2}$-inch cubes.

2. Steam 12–15 minutes or until tender.

3. Rinse to cool and let stand.

4. In a large bowl, combine all other ingredients and mix well.

5. Toss in potatoes and mix; chill for at least 45 minutes before serving.

&. FANCY FRUIT SALAD

Total yield: 9 servings or 4 1/2 C
Serving size: 1/2 C
Each serving provides:
Calories: 97
Protein: 1.73 grams
Fat: 0.2 gram
Carbohydrate: 22.07 grams

1 can pineapple tidbits, packed in its own juice, 20 ounces

1 1/2 T cornstarch

3/4 C plain nonfat yogurt

2 tsp granulated fructose

1/2 tsp vanilla extract

1/4 tsp almond extract

1 small (5-inch) banana, sliced

1 C seedless red grapes, halved

1 medium peach, sliced, pitted, and cut into chunks

1 C fresh strawberries, sliced

1. Drain pineapple juice into medium saucepan.

2. Add cornstarch to juice; stir to dissolve.

3. Heat juice over medium heat until thick and bubbly, stirring constantly.

4. Remove from heat and cool 15–20 minutes.

5. Add yogurt, fructose, and extracts; stir well with a wire whisk.

6. Place all fruit in large bowl. Pour sauce over fruit; stir to combine.

7. Cover salad and chill for 3 hours before serving.

Use as a lunch, brunch, or dinner salad.

⚛ HOT PASTA SALAD

Serve as a side salad.

Total yield: 4 servings
Serving size: approximately 1 C
Each serving provides:
Calories: 190
Protein: 6.54 grams
Fat: 1.9 grams
Carbohydrate: 36.69 grams

1 medium green bell pepper,
cut into $1/4$-inch strips

$1/2$ medium red onion,
cut into thin slices

2 T prepared Butter Buds

2 tsp poppy seeds

3 C cooked spaghetti (6 ounces dry semolina)

1 large tomato, sliced into thin wedges

1. In a microwave-safe bowl, combine all ingredients, except spaghetti and tomato wedges.

2. Microwave 3–5 minutes on high, stirring once.

3. Add spaghetti and tomato wedges and toss.

4. Microwave on medium setting an additional 2–3 minutes.

5. Let stand, covered, for 1 minute. Serve.

ℛ HURRY CURRY SALAD

This is a main meal salad.

Total yield: 2 servings
Serving size: 1 main meal salad
Each serving provides:
Calories: 235 (includes ¹/₄ C dressing)
Protein: 25.7 grams
Fat: 3.5 grams
Carbohydrate: 25.18 grams

iceberg lettuce for two
(approximately 4 C)

16 slices water chestnuts

1 stalk celery, diced

4–6 large mushrooms, sliced

2 green onions, chopped

1 C Quick Cooked Chicken (p. 142), diced

¹/₂ tomato, chopped

2 T raisins

¹/₂ C Creamy Curry Dressing (p. 3)

1. Dress two meal plates with desired amount of lettuce.
2. In a bowl, toss together water chestnuts, celery, mushrooms, and green onions.
3. Divide equally and place on top of lettuce.
4. Place ¹/₂ C chicken on top of each salad.
5. Top each salad with raisins and tomatoes.
6. Top each salad with ¹/₄ C Creamy Curry Dressing and serve.

◈ SEATTLE SALAD

An out-of-towner's favorite

Total yield: 2 servings or 4 C
Serving size: 2 C
Each serving provides:
Calories: 332
Protein: 24.73 grams
Fat: 7.6 grams
Carbohydrate: 41.17 grams

$^1/_2$ medium red apple, diced into small bits

2 tsp lemon juice

1 can lowfat pink salmon, 6.5 ounces

1 C cooked wild rice

$^1/_2$ C celery, diced

1 T green onion, chopped

2 T raisins

2 tsp pine nuts

$^1/_3$ C of your favorite oil-free creamy Italian dressing

1 tsp Dijon mustard

$^1/_4$ tsp dill weed

1. Put apple bits into bowl and sprinkle with lemon juice.

2. Stir and let stand 5 minutes.

3. Add all remaining ingredients; toss.

4. Chill before serving.

Serve with 1 C Emerald City Soup (p. 105).

⟲ SHRIMP-ATIZER SALAD

A sensational summer luncheon salad.

Total yield: 4 servings
Serving size: 1 side salad
Each serving provides:
Calories: 123
Protein: 24.67 grams
Fat: 1.9 grams
Carbohydrate: 1.8 grams

$3/4$ pound cooked shrimp

$3/4$ C celery, diced

$1/2$ C red bell pepper, diced

$1/4$ C 1 percent cottage cheese

2 T plain nonfat yogurt

1 tsp nonfat milk

1 small clove garlic, pressed

2 tsp Dijon mustard

$1/2$ tsp lemon juice

$1/4$ tsp each crushed basil, oregano, and tarragon leaves

$1/8$ tsp black pepper

4 butter lettuce leaves

1. In a mixing bowl, toss together shrimp, celery, and bell pepper.

2. In a small mixing bowl, combine all other ingredients, except lettuce; beat with electric mixer until smooth.

3. Pour sauce over shrimp/vegetable mixture and toss to combine; chill 30–45 minutes. Place lettuce leaves on 4 salad plates and chill.

4. Spoon 4 equal portions of salad onto leaves and serve.

✑ "SWEET-HOTS" SALAD

Total yield: 2 servings or 2 ¹/₂ C
Serving size: 1 ¹/₄ C
Each serving provides:
Calories: 56
Protein: 1.35 grams
Fat: 0
Carbohydrate: 12.65 grams

1 ¹/₂ C grated carrots

1 C grated red cabbage

1 ¹/₂ T diet maple syrup

1 T lemon juice

2 pinches ground red pepper

1. In a bowl, combine carrots and cabbage.

2. In another small bowl, combine remaining ingredients and mix well.

3. Pour "sweet-hots" sauce over cabbage and carrot mixture; toss well.

4. Chill *slightly* before serving.

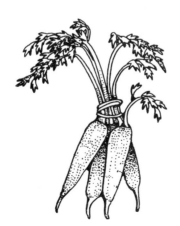

Chapter 5

SOUPS
AND
STEWS

Soups and Stews

Coldcumber Soup

Chowderhead Soup

Cream of Mushroom Soup

Emerald City Soup

Heartwarming Chili

Hearty Stew

Seafood Corn Chowder

Speedy French Onion Soup

Mary's Winter Stew

Wayne's Chicken Soup
for Several

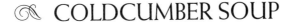 COLDCUMBER SOUP

A perfect summer soup!

Total yield: 2 servings
Serving size: 1 C
Each serving provides:
Calories: 54
Protein: 5.16 grams
Fat: trace (0.2 gram total/recipe)
Carbohydrate: 8.12 grams

1 English cucumber, peeled and
sliced (approximately 1 pound)

$3/4$ C plain nonfat yogurt

1 packet (5.5 grams) low-sodium
instant chicken broth

$1/4$ C fresh cilantro, chopped

1 tsp white wine vinegar (champagne vinegar preferred)

1. Combine all ingredients in a blender; blend until smooth.

2. Serve chilled.

Serve with your favorite sandwich.

ᘓ CHOWDERHEAD SOUP

Total yield: 8 servings or 10 1/2 C
Serving size: approximately 1 1/3 C
Each serving provides:
Calories: 169
Protein: 14.41 grams
Fat: 1.3 grams
Carbohydrate: 24.91 grams

3 C water

2 medium white potatoes,
cut into 1-inch cubes

1 large onion, peeled and diced

1 C celery, chopped

1 tsp dried thyme

1/4 rounded tsp pepper

2 bay leaves

1/2 pound halibut, cut into 1/2-inch chunks

2 (6.5-ounce) cans clams in juice

1/4 C white wine

1 1/2 C nonfat milk

1/3 C nonfat powdered milk

2 tsp dried parsley

1/8 tsp Tabasco sauce

1. In 4 1/2- to 5-quart dutch oven, combine water, potatoes, onion, celery, and spices.

2. Cover and bring to boil.

3. Reduce heat to medium; simmer for 12 minutes.

4. Add clams with their juice, halibut chunks, and wine.

5. Reduce heat to low and simmer covered for 15 minutes. *Do not boil.*

6. Combine powdered and liquid milks; mix until dissolved and add to soup.

7. Cover and simmer soup 15 more minutes. *Do not boil.*

8. Remove bay leaves and season with Tabasco sauce.

9. Garnish with parsley and serve.

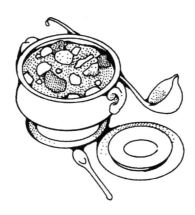

CREAM OF MUSHROOM SOUP

Total yield: 2 servings or 3 C
Serving size: 1 1/2 C
Each serving provides:
Calories: 90
Protein: 5.21 grams
Fat: trace (0.4 gram total/recipe)
Carbohydrate: 16.84 grams

2 C water combined with 1 T defatted
Sona English Style Beef Tea concentrate
(or 1 bouillon cube)

1/4 rounded tsp poultry seasoning

2 C fresh mushrooms, sliced

2 1/2 T farina or Cream of Wheat

3 T nonfat powdered milk

1. In a medium saucepan, combine beef tea mixture, poultry seasoning, and mushrooms.
2. Bring to rolling boil; reduce heat to medium-low.
3. Cover and cook 7 minutes.
4. Sprinkle farina into pan and stir to combine.
5. Cover and cook 7 minutes more, stirring occasionally.
6. Remove from heat and pour mixture into a blender.
7. Sprinkle powdered milk gradually into blender.
8. Purée until smooth and serve.

For a thicker mushroom "gravy," add 1 more tablespoon of powdered milk.

⌀ EMERALD CITY SOUP

Total yield: 2 servings or 3 C
Serving size: 1 1/2 C
Each serving provides:
Calories: 66
Protein: 5.47 grams
Fat: 0.3 gram
Carbohydrate: 10.36 grams

6 C sliced zucchini
(approximately 1 1/2 pounds)

1/8 tsp salt

1. Steam zucchini for 10–12 minutes, until soft.

2. Place zucchini in blender and add salt.

3. Blend until smooth (approximately 1 minute).

4. Hot water may be added during blending process to achieve a desired serving consistency.

5. Serve immediately.

Garnish with fresh ground pepper, red apple slices, or 1 percent cottage cheese.

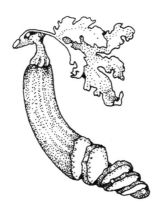

ᘒ HEARTWARMING CHILI

Total yield: 6 servings or 11 C
Serving size: 1 ³/₄ C
Each serving provides:
Calories: 240
Protein: 13.67 grams
Fat: 1.5 grams
Carbohydrate: 42.96 grams

1 medium red onion, chopped

4–6 cloves garlic, coarsely chopped

16 ounces mild salsa*

2 tsp ground cumin

1 tsp chili powder*

4 C tomato juice*

2 large green bell peppers, chopped

1 medium/large red or gold bell pepper, chopped

1 C cooked kidney beans (8.5-ounce can)*

2 C cooked black beans (15-ounce can)*

¹/₂ C raw cracked bulgur

¹/₃ C minced fresh cilantro

¹/₃ C frozen corn

1. In a 4 ¹/₂- to 5-quart dutch oven, combine onion, garlic, salsa, spices, and tomato juice. Simmer 10 minutes on medium-low heat.

2. Add peppers and beans; simmer 15 minutes. Stir in bulgur; simmer for 15 more minutes, stirring frequently.

3. Add cilantro and frozen corn; stir well and remove from heat. Cover and let stand 15 minutes before serving.

Serve with Tija's Favorite Cornbread (p. 68).
*Choose low-sodium and low-sugar brands.

SOUPS AND STEWS

⟡ HEARTY STEW

Total yield: 6 servings or approximately 10 C
Serving size: 1 ²/₃ C
Each serving provides:
Calories: 206
Protein: 14.91 grams
Fat: 3 grams
Carbohydrate: 29.84 grams

3 C cold water

¹/₄ C lite soy sauce

2 cloves garlic, minced

2 bay leaves

¹/₂ tsp thyme

¹/₄ tsp pepper

2 medium onions, thinly sliced

2 stalks celery, diced

2 medium potatoes, cut into 1-inch chunks

2 carrots, chopped

8 mushrooms, sliced

³/₄ pound ground turkey (93 percent fat free),
browned and drained

3 T cornstarch

1. In a 4 ¹/₂- to 5-quart dutch oven, combine all ingredients, except turkey and cornstarch.

2. Bring mixture to boil; reduce heat and cover, simmering 45–60 minutes.

3. Remove bay leaves; stir in browned turkey.

4. Dissolve cornstarch in ¹/₂ C cold water and slowly add to stew, stirring until thick. Serve hot.

ℭ SEAFOOD CORN CHOWDER

Total yield: 4 servings or 6 C
Serving size: 1 ¹/₂ C
Each serving provides:
Calories: 175
Protein: 18.52 grams
Fat: 2.4 grams
Carbohydrate: 19.83 grams

2 C thawed frozen corn (reserve 1 C)

1 C low-sodium chicken broth

¹/₂ C nonfat milk

¹/₈ tsp black pepper

1 (10-ounce) can whole baby clams, drained (or 5 ounces dry)

8 ounces natural clam juice

1 C red bell pepper, diced

1 C fresh mushrooms, sliced

8 ounces medium bay scallops, raw

paprika to garnish individual servings

1. Combine 1 C corn, broth, milk, and pepper in a small saucepan; bring to boil.

2. Reduce heat to low and cook for 5 minutes.

3. Pour mixture into blender; blend at highest setting for 20 seconds.

4. Pour mixture through a strainer into a large saucepan, discarding corn shells.

5. Add remaining ingredients, including reserved corn, to pan and return to boil.

6. Reduce heat to low, cover, and cook 10–12 minutes, stirring occasionally.

7. Serve hot, garnished with paprika.

∽ SPEEDY FRENCH ONION SOUP

Total yield: 4 servings or 6 C
Serving size: 1 ¹/₂ C
Each serving provides:
Calories: 87
Protein: 3.72 grams
Fat: 1.9 grams
Carbohydrate: 13.75 grams

> 3 medium sweet onions, peeled and sliced (approximately 3 C)
>
> ¹/₃ C prepared Butter Buds
>
> 2 pinches black pepper
>
> 3 C prepared defatted Sona English Style Beef Tea concentrate
>
> 1 C water
>
> 1 T Worcestershire sauce
>
> 3 T grated Parmesan cheese

1. In a 3-quart microwave-safe dish, combine onions, Butter Buds, and pepper.

2. Cover and cook in microwave on high for 8 minutes.

3. Stir in broth, water, and Worcestershire sauce.

4. Cover and cook on high for another 8 minutes.

5. Stir and cook on medium setting for 10 minutes more.

6. Remove from microwave and let stand 5 minutes, covered, to continue final cooking.

7. Sprinkle with Parmesan cheese and serve.

Serve with Farmer's French Bread (p. 78).

ᏇᎿ MARY'S WINTER STEW

For those cold winter nights!

Total yield: 9 servings or 18 C
Serving size: 2 C
Each serving provides:
Calories: 177
Protein: 8.57 grams
Fat: 2.3 grams
Carbohydrate: 30.5 grams

1 medium eggplant, cut into 1-inch chunks

salt

9 cups coarsely chopped greens
(kale, spinach, or mustard)

5 ¹/₂ C flavored broth, chicken or vegetable
(8 packets instant)

2 (28-ounce) cans Italian plum tomatoes, undrained

1 C dry red wine

4 carrots, coarsely chopped

1 large red onion, coarsely chopped

2 celery stalks, coarsely chopped

2 medium red bell peppers, coarsely chopped

6 medium garlic cloves, coarsely chopped

4 fresh parsley sprigs

1 T dried sweet basil

1 T crushed dried oregano

1 tsp dried rosemary

2 bay leaves

2 C rolled oats

fresh ground pepper

1. Place eggplant in colander and sprinkle with salt; let stand 30 minutes.

2. Rinse and pat dry.

3. In an 8-quart dutch oven, combine greens, flavored broth, tomatoes, and wine; bring to boil.

4. Add eggplant and all remaining ingredients, except oats and pepper.

5. Reduce heat, cover and simmer until tender, about 30 minutes, stirring occasionally to break up tomatoes.

6. Stir in oats; cover and simmer an additional 10 minutes.

7. Discard bay leaves and parsley.

8. Let stand 30 minutes to thicken.

9. Season with pepper to taste, and serve with One-Hour Oat Bread (p. 69).

This recipe was adapted from a Bon Appétit original recipe in the November 1989 issue.

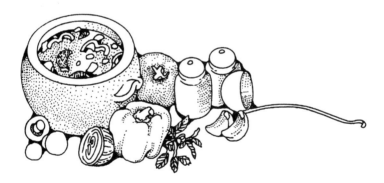

℘ WAYNE'S CHICKEN SOUP FOR SEVERAL

Total yield: 10 servings
Serving size: 2 C
Each serving provides:
Calories: 248
Protein: 33.13 grams
Fat: 4.9 grams*
Carbohydrates: 17.85 grams

5 quarts water

3 skinless, boneless chicken breasts
(approximately 3 pounds)

1 C raw brown rice

2 C celery, chopped

2 large carrots, chopped

$^1/_2$ pound fresh mushrooms, sliced (3 C)

6 green onions, chopped

2 T chicken bouillon (no salt added)

1. In an 8-quart dutch oven, bring 3 quarts water to boil.
2. Add chicken breasts and boil until cooked through (meat should not be pink).
3. Remove chicken and shred meat.
4. Return shredded meat to dutch oven; add rice and vegetables, and 2 quarts additional water.

*More fat can be removed by refrigerating soup and skimming fat off the top after it has chilled!

5. Bring to boil, stirring constantly.

6. Reduce heat to simmer (low) and stir in bouillon.

7. Cover; cook 1 $1/2$ hours, stirring occasionally.

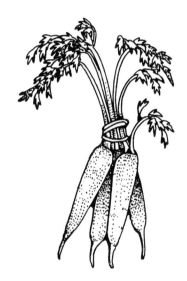

Chapter 6

SIDE CARS

Side Cars

Shrimp Cocktail

ɪ POTATOES

Baked Potato
Potato "Dress-Ups"!
Pronto Potato
Baked Potato Chips
Mashed Potato Magic
Potatoes Au Gratia
Perfect Pasta

RICE AND GRAINS ɪ

Basic Brown Rice
Quick Carbs for Two
Raisin-Orange Pilaf
"Wild-Style" Stuffing
Wild Rice Medley

VEGGIES ɪ

Spicy Yams
Stuffed Acorn Squash
Butter Onions
Roasted Cinnamon Corn
Roasted Bell Peppers
Simply Wonderful
Veggies

⚘ SHRIMP COCKTAIL

Total yield: 2 servings
Serving size: 6 shrimp
Each serving provides:
Calories: 190
Protein: 30.69 grams
Fat: 1.5 grams
Carbohydrate: 13.44 grams

12 cooked tiger shrimp

$^1/_2$ C low-calorie catsup

$^1/_4$ C low-salt tomato sauce

2 T lemon juice

1 T lime juice

2 T green onion, minced

1 tsp Worcestershire sauce

2 $^1/_2$ tsp prepared horseradish
(not creamed)

$^1/_2$ tsp chili powder, salt free

butter or romaine lettuce leaves

1. In a blender, combine all ingredients, except shrimp and lettuce; blend until smooth.

2. Divide sauce into two small glass bowls and chill.

3. Dress two salad plates with lettuce leaves.

4. Place 6 cooked shrimp over lettuce on each plate.

5. Serve prawns with sauce.

⁊ BAKED POTATO

Total yield: 1 serving
Serving size: 1 medium potato
Each serving provides:
Calories: 145
Protein: 3 grams
Fat: 0.2 gram
Carbohydrate: 32.8 grams

1 medium potato

1. Preheat oven to 350°F.

2. Wash and scrub potato.

3. Poke holes in potato with fork, and wrap potato in aluminum foil.

4. Bake for one hour, or until done.

5. Remove from oven and unwrap.

6. Slice potato open by cutting an X in top.

7. Dress it up any way you like from suggestions in Potato "Dress-ups!" (p. 119).

For a faster potato, see Pronto Potato (p. 120).

◯ POTATO "DRESS-UPS"!

This page is dedicated to fun potatoes made your way.
Try various combinations of the ingredients below on your
baked potato.

Total yield: 1/4 C (plus potato)
Serving size: 1/4 C (plus potato)
Each serving provides:
Calories: 145 plus your choice of dress-ups below
Protein: 3 grams
Fat: 0.2 gram
Carbohydrate: 32.8 grams

1 medium potato, baked

Choose your favorite dress-up:

1/4 C prepared Butter Buds, 24 calories

1/4 C My Best Barbecue Sauce (p. 17), 44 calories

1/4 C 1 percent cottage cheese, 45 calories

1/4 C Beef Gravy (p. 13), 14 calories

1/4 C Mock Mayo (p. 28), 40 calories

1/4 C Tex Mex Salsa (p. 11), 16 calories

1/4 C plain nonfat yogurt, 23 calories

1/4 C Heartwarming Chili (p. 106), 40 calories

1/4 Veggie Dip (p. 8), 40 calories

PRONTO POTATO

For those who want it NOW!

Total yield: 1 serving
Serving size: 1 medium potato
Each serving provides:
Calories: 145
Protein: 3 grams
Fat: 0.2 gram
Carbohydrate: 32.8 grams

1 medium potato

1. Wash and scrub potato, pat dry.

2. Prick skin with a fork several times to allow moisture to escape during cooking.

3. Place in a microwave-safe bowl and loosely cover with plastic wrap or paper towel.

4. Microwave on high 5–6 minutes, turning one time, mid-cycle.

5. For each extra potato cooked at the same time, add 4 minutes.

6. Remove from microwave; wait about 4 minutes (microwaved food continues to cook for a few minutes after being removed from a microwave oven); test for doneness.

To top, see Potato "Dress-Ups!" (p. 119).

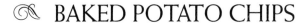 # BAKED POTATO CHIPS

The french fry alternative.

Total yield: 2 servings
Serving size: ¹/₂ potato made into chips
Each serving provides:
Calories: 122
Protein: 1.53 grams
Fat: 0.1 gram
Carbohydrate: 28.74 grams

1 large raw white potato

1 tsp garlic powder

2 T dry Butter Buds

pinch ground white pepper (optional)

1. Preheat oven to broil.

2. Slice potato into very thin round "chips."

3. Lay on nonstick baking sheet.

4. Sprinkle half of the Butter Buds and garlic powder over potato slices.

5. Lightly sprinkle a pinch of ground pepper over potatoes.

6. Broil 4–5 minutes or until potato slices bubble and turn brown (be careful not to burn them).

7. Remove from oven, turn potato slices over, and repeat the seasoning process.

8. Broil an additional 1–3 minutes; serve.

Serve with low-sodium, low-calorie catsup. This is a great side dish for chicken recipes.

℞ MASHED POTATO MAGIC

Total yield: 4 servings or 4 $1/2$ C
Serving size: 1 $1/8$ C
Each serving provides:
Calories: 130
Protein: 3.79 grams
Fat: 0.15 gram
Carbohydrate: 28.37 grams

3 medium potatoes

$1/2$ C nonfat milk, at room temperature

3 T warm water

1 $1/2$ T lite soy sauce

1 tsp dried minced onion flakes

1 tsp dried parsley flakes

$1/4$ tsp garlic powder

dry Butter Buds to taste

Traditional method:

1. Peel potatoes and cut into small pieces.

2. Steam until tender.

3. Place potatoes in large mixing bowl and mash.

4. Add all ingredients except water and Butter Buds.

5. Whip until fluffy with an electric mixer.

6. Add water as needed, by tablespoons, to achieve desired consistency.

7. Serve, sprinkling Butter Buds to taste.

Quick method:

1. Cook potatoes in microwave (see Pronto Potato, p. 120).
   Do not peel.

2. Slice potatoes into small pieces.

3. Place all ingredients but potatoes, water, and Butter Buds in blender.

4. Add potatoes, blending slowly.

5. Add water as needed, by tablespoons, to achieve desired consistency. Periodically scrape potatoes down from sides of blender.

6. Spoon potatoes from blender to serving dish.

7. Serve, sprinkling Butter Buds to taste.

Great with Herbed Chicken (p. 147).

ᘏ POTATOES AU GRATIA

Total yield: 4 servings
Serving size: 2 1/2-by-2 1/2-inch slice
Each serving provides:
Calories: 135
Protein: 3.67 grams
Fat: 0.5 gram
Carbohydrate: 28.96 grams

2 large (5-inch) russet potatoes

1 C red onion, sliced

2 tsp salt-free dill herb mix*

1/2 C sliced mushrooms

2 T whole wheat flour

1 C low-sodium beef bouillon (1 packet or cube)

1. Spray a microwave-safe casserole dish with nonstick cooking spray.

2. Slice potatoes and onions thinly (1/4 inch thick or less).

3. Cover bottom of prepared dish with half of potatoes; place half of the onion slices over potato layer; sprinkle 1 tsp of dill herb mix and 1 T of flour over top.

4. Layer remaining potatoes, onions, and sliced mushrooms, ending with mushrooms.

5. Sprinkle remaining dill herb mix and flour over mushrooms; pour bouillon into edge of dish, carefully avoiding herbs and flour.

6. Loosely cover dish with plastic wrap and microwave on high for 12 minutes.

7. Set oven on broil; after removing plastic wrap, place dish in oven on highest rack and broil 3–5 minutes until onion edges turn brown. Remove from the oven and serve.

Commercially available in your grocery store's spice section.

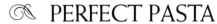 PERFECT PASTA

Total yield: 4 servings or 8 C
Serving size: 2 C
Each serving provides:
Calories: 226
Protein: 9.06 grams
Fat: 2.3 grams
Carbohydrate: 42.27 grams

olive oil cooking spray

$^{1}/_{2}$ C onions, diced

1 C broccoli, chopped fine

1 each red and yellow bell pepper, chopped fine

1 medium clove garlic, minced

1 medium tomato, chopped

$^{1}/_{2}$ C fresh parsley, chopped

4 tsp fresh basil, chopped

2 T low-sodium chicken broth

4 C cooked spinach or garden spiral pasta (8 ounces dry)

1 T fresh grated Parmesan cheese

1. Spray skillet with olive oil cooking spray.

2. Saute onions, broccoli, bell peppers, and garlic in prepared nonstick skillet for 6 minutes over low heat until veggies. are tender. Stir in tomato, cooking 4 more minutes.

3. In a small bowl, combine parsley, basil, and chicken broth, mixing well.

4. Spray cooked pasta noodles with olive oil cooking spray for 4 seconds and toss lightly.

5. Add veggies and broth mixture.

6. Toss well, chill. Sprinkle with Parmesan cheese before serving.

🖎 BASIC BROWN RICE

Total yield: 4 servings or 2 C
Serving size: ¹/₂ C
Each serving provides:
Calories: 110
Protein: 2.95 grams
Fat: 0.6 gram
Carbohydrate: 23.2 grams

1 ²/₃ C water

²/₃ C raw brown rice

1. In a medium saucepan, combine water and rice.
2. Bring to a rolling boil.
3. Reduce heat to low, cover, and simmer 50 minutes, or until all liquid is absorbed.
4. Remove from heat *(do not stir rice)* and let stand, covered, for 10 minutes.
5. Fluff with fork before serving, or allow to cool and store in refrigerator.

⟡ QUICK CARBS FOR TWO

Total yield: 2 servings or 2 C
Serving size: 1 C
Each serving provides:
Calories: 175
Protein: 4.93 grams
Fat: 0.1 gram
Carbohydrate: 38.6 grams

1 C water

$^1/_3$ C raw cracked bulgur

2 T dry Butter Buds

1 tsp dry instant broth, low sodium (chicken or beef)

3 T couscous

1. Place all ingredients in a 1-quart saucepan and cover.
2. Bring to boil; reduce heat and simmer on low 10–12 minutes.
3. Fluff with a fork and serve.

RAISIN-ORANGE PILAF

Total yield: 2 servings, approximately 1 ²/₃ C
Serving size: approximately ³/₄ C
Each serving provides:
Calories: 194
Protein: 4.71 grams
Fat: trace
Carbohydrate: 43.74 grams

¹/₂ C water

¹/₂ C orange juice

¹/₂ C raw cracked bulgur

1 T raisins, minced

1 tsp lite soy sauce

¹/₂ tsp grated orange peel

1. In a 1-quart saucepan, combine all ingredients.
2. Cover, bring to boil; reduce heat and simmer for 15 minutes, until tender.
3. Serve immediately.

This makes a quick luncheon dish, or serve with Glazed Tender-loins with Blackberry Sauce (p. 150).

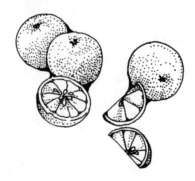

"WILD-STYLE" STUFFING

No bird necessary!

Total yield: 4 servings or 4 C
Serving size: 1 C
Each serving provides:
Calories: 170
Protein: 5.17 grams
Fat: 0.5 gram
Carbohydrate: 36.2 grams

2 C water combined with 1 T defatted
Sona English Style Beef Tea concentrate

$^3/_4$ C raw cracked bulgur

$^1/_4$ C wild rice

$^1/_2$ C celery, diced

$^1/_4$ C onion, chopped

$^1/_4$ C red bell pepper, chopped

1 T orange juice concentrate

$^1/_4$ tsp grated orange rind

1. Combine all ingredients in a 2-quart saucepan.

2. Cover, bring to boil; reduce heat and simmer 30–35 minutes, stirring occasionally.

3. Serve immediately.

ℭℛ WILD RICE MEDLEY

Total yield: 4 servings
Serving size: 1 C
Each serving provides:
Calories: 189
Protein: 7.9 grams
Fat: 0.5 gram
Carbohydrate: 38.23 grams

2 C water

1 C wild rice

$^3/_4$ C celery, chopped

1 C fresh mushrooms, sliced

$^3/_4$ C red bell pepper, diced

3 T green onion, chopped

$^1/_2$ red apple, chopped

$^1/_2$ C pineapple tidbits

1 $^1/_2$ C defatted chicken broth

1 T lite soy sauce

1. Preheat oven to 350°F.

2. Combine water and rice in saucepan, bring to boil; cover and simmer 20 minutes. Remove from heat and drain water.

3. Toss rice with celery, mushrooms, bell pepper, onion, apples, and pineapple. Place in a 2-quart casserole dish.

4. Combine broth and soy sauce and pour into dish.

5. Cover loosely with foil; bake one hour.

6. Remove from oven and drain off any excess liquids; mix and serve.

Serve with fish, turkey, or chicken.

ᔭ SPICY YAMS

Total yield: 4 servings or 4 C
Serving size: 1 C
Each serving provides:
Calories: 160
Protein: 2.03 grams
Fat: 0.3 gram
Carbohydrate: 37.3 grams

2 large (6-inch) yams (3 C cooked)

$^1/_4$ tsp cinnamon

$^1/_8$ tsp nutmeg

$^1/_8$ tsp allspice

2 T orange juice concentrate

$^1/_4$ C raisins, minced

1. Preheat oven to 350°F.
2. Wrap yams in aluminum foil and bake for 1 $^1/_2$ hours.
3. Remove foil and skins from yams.
4. Place in mixing bowl; add remaining ingredients, except raisins.
5. Whip with electric mixer until fluffy.
6. Stir in raisins in by hand.
7. Spoon mixture into a nonstick 2-quart casserole dish; smooth evenly.
8. Return to oven, and bake uncovered for 12–15 minutes more. Serve warm.

A perfect accompaniment for turkey.

⚮ STUFFED ACORN SQUASH

Total yield: 2 servings
Serving size: half squash
Each serving provides:
Calories: 142
Protein: 2.13 grams
Fat: 0.6 gram
Carbohydrate: 32.02 grams

1 medium acorn squash (2 pounds)

1 ripe D'Anjou pear (or your favorite apple)

1 ¹/₂ T cinnamon

1. Cut off top of squash and spoon out seeds and pulp.

2. Remove core from pear; dice into small bits.

3. Fill squash with pear and sprinkle cinnamon into center.

4. Place squash in a microwave-safe bowl; loosely cover with plastic wrap.

5. Microwave on high setting for 12 minutes, or until tender (based on 6 minutes per pound of squash).

6. Remove squash, slice in half, and distribute pear evenly over halves.

7. Serve hot.

SIDE CARS

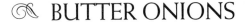 BUTTER ONIONS

This is a wonderful side dish for fish and poultry.

Total yield: 2 servings
Serving size: 1 onion
Each serving provides:
Calories: 66
Protein: 1.72 grams
Fat: 0.2 gram
Carbohydrate: 14.33 grams

> 2 medium sweet onions, unpeeled
>
> 1/4 C prepared Butter Buds*
>
> dill weed, dried

1. Cut tops off onions, but do not peel.

2. Place onions in a 1-quart microwave-safe dish; loosely cover with plastic wrap.

3. Microwave on high setting for 8 1/2 minutes *(add 60–90 seconds for each additional onion; one onion requires 7 minutes of cooking time)*.

4. Carefully remove plastic wrap and cut an X on top of each onion.

5. Pour 2 T Butter Buds into each onion and sprinkle with dill weed to taste.

*You may substitute Fresh Veggie Dip (p. 8) for the Butter Buds.

ℛ ROASTED CINNAMON CORN

Total yield: 6 servings or 6 ears
Serving size: 1 ear of corn
Each serving provides:
Calories: 90
Protein: 2.78 grams
Fat: 0.9 gram
Carbohydrate: 17.7 grams

1 ($^1/_2$-ounce) package dry Butter Buds

$^1/_4$ tsp cinnamon (or your favorite crushed herb)

6 medium ears sweet corn, in husks

cinnamon, to sprinkle

1. In a small bowl or glass dish, combine dry Butter Buds and $^1/_4$ tsp cinnamon; add $^1/_2$ C boiling water and stir until dissolved.

2. Place in refrigerator and allow to chill and thicken (4 hours).

3. Remove outer layer of corn husk on each ear, and tear husks into long strips. Peel back remaining husk layers from ears, being careful not to break them from cobs.

4. Remove all inner silk and lightly sprinkle each ear with cinnamon.

5. Pull husks back up over ears and tie off husk ends with torn husk strips, securing tightly. Soak corn for 5–10 minutes in a sink filled with cold water.

6. Remove and place corn on hot barbecue or outdoor grill; roast for 20 minutes, turning every 5 minutes to roast evenly. Remove from grill and peel back husks.

7. Brush ears with chilled cinnamon butter and serve. Use remaining butter for dipping.

⌒ ROASTED BELL PEPPERS

Total yield: 4 servings
Serving size: 1 pepper
Each serving provides:
Calories: 24
Protein: 1.55 grams
Fat: 0.4 gram
Carbohydrate: 3.55 grams

4 red bell peppers
(or your favorite colored peppers)

1. Preheat oven to broil.
2. Place whole peppers on rack of broiler pan.
3. Broil about 3 inches from heat, turning every 5 minutes for 20 minutes (until charred).
4. Place peppers in bowl and cover, so that peppers will steam until cool.
5. Peel peppers, starting from bottom.
6. Cut off tops, discard seeds and lining.

Serve this versatile vegetable with any meal.

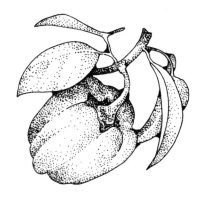

ℛ SIMPLY WONDERFUL VEGGIES

Total yield: 4 servings
Serving size: approximately 1 C
Each serving provides:
Calories: 36
Protein: 1.91 grams
Fat: 0.3 gram
Carbohydrate: 6.41 grams

1 C broccoli, chopped

1 red bell pepper, cut in thin strips

1 carrot, sliced thin

$^1/_2$ medium white onion, sliced in rings

2 stalks celery, cut into chunks

1 T dried cilantro

1. Place veggies in 2-quart microwave-safe dish and toss.
2. Sprinkle cilantro over veggies.
3. Loosely cover dish with plastic wrap.
4. Cook on high 4–5 minutes until tender.
5. Serve immediately.

MICROWAVING
VEGETABLES ᔧ ᔧ ᔧ ᔧ ᔧ

Microwaving is a great way to cook vegetables. Vegetables retain their color, taste, and nutrients better when microwaved than when prepared with most other cooking methods.

Cook your vegetables in a round dish loosely covered with a lid or plastic wrap. Square and rectangular dishes tend to overcook foods, as microwaves concentrate in corners.

Microwaves cook from the outside of a dish first. Arrange any thick or dense slices around the outer edge of the dish. Thin slices will cook faster and should be placed toward the center of the dish. If possible, cut the vegetables into similar sizes to ensure even cooking.

Cooking time varies greatly based on the amount of vegetables in the microwave. If you double the volume of food in a recipe, your cooking time will be much longer.

When you finish cooking your vegetables, remove plastic wrap by pulling back the side that is *away* from you first. This allows hot

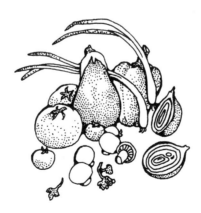

Chapter 7

ENTRÉES

Entrées

❧ CHICKEN

Two Easy

Quick Cooked
Chicken

Broiled Barbecued
Chicken

Chicken Elegance

Chicken Parmesan

Easy Skillet Chicken

Herbed Chicken

Chicken for Two

Teriyaki Chicken

❧ TURKEY

Glazed Tenderloins with
Blackberry Sauce

Ground Turkey
Spaghetti Sauce

Turkey-Stuffed Peppers

SEAFOOD ❧

Italian Fish

Oriental Fish

Fish à l'Orange

Breaded Fillets

Crab-Stuffed Oranges

Halibut Steaks with
Wine Sauce

Shrimp Primavera

Sweet and Sour Prawns
with Couscous

BURGERS AND MEATLOAVES ❧

Better Burgers

Mushroom and
Onion Burgers

Cheese Meatloaf

Meet My Meatloaf

🐦 TWO EASY

A tangy poultry marinade.

Total yield: marinates 1 pound of poultry breasts
Serving size: 1 recipe
Each serving provides:
Calories: 164
Protein: 1.25 grams
Fat: 0.3 gram
Carbohydrate: 39.08 grams

1 pound poultry

2 T water

2 T lemon juice

2 T lime juice

2 T honey

2 tsp lite soy sauce

2 tsp dry cooking sherry

2 small cloves garlic,
minced (about 1 tsp)

1. Cut 1 pound of your favorite poultry breasts into quarter sections.

2. Place poultry in durable plastic bag.

3. In a small bowl, combine remaining ingredients to make a marinade; stir until honey dissolves.

4. Pour marinade into plastic bag; seal bag tightly, releasing most of air.

5. Place bag in refrigerator 4–16 hours (or overnight).

6. Broil poultry on top oven rack for 12–15 minutes turning once; baste with reserve marinade.

7. Serve poultry with cooked marinade juice.

QUICK COOKED CHICKEN

Designed to save you time when preparing recipes that call for cooked chicken, such as chicken salads or crepes.

Total yield: 4 servings
Serving size: ¹/₄ pound
Each serving provides:
Calories: 142
Protein: 28.52 grams
Fat: 3.1 grams
Carbohydrate: 0

1 pound skinless, boneless chicken,
cut into strips

1. Arrange chicken in a microwave-safe dish, placing thickest strips on the outside.

2. Cover dish with plastic wrap.

3. Microwave on high for 6 minutes, turning chicken once after 3 minutes.

4. Make a slit in chicken to check doneness; meat should be neither pink nor rubbery.

❧ BROILED BARBECUED CHICKEN

Total yield: 4 servings
Serving size: 2 strips
Each serving provides:
Calories: 186
Protein: 28.42 grams
Fat: 3.2 grams
Carbohydrate: 10.88 grams

> 2 skinless, boneless chicken breasts,
> cut into 8 strips
>
> 1 C My Best Barbecue Sauce (p. 17)

1. Baste chicken strips with barbecue sauce.

2. Place chicken on broiler pan and set on top rack of oven (4–5 inches from broiling unit).

3. Broil until browned on top side.

4. Turn and baste; broil until browned all over.

5. Serve, using remaining sauce for dipping.

Serve with a baked potato; see Potato "Dress-Ups"! (p. 119).

ℰ CHICKEN ELEGANCE

A taste of France in 30 minutes.

Total yield: 4 servings
Serving size: half breast
Each serving provides:
Calories: 195 grams
Protein: 27.85 grams
Fat: 3.3 grams
Carbohydrate: 13.48 grams

2 skinless, boneless chicken breasts,
cut into halves

$^1/_8$ tsp salt

1 $^1/_2$ C sliced mushrooms

1 C water

$^1/_2$ C fruity white wine

$^1/_2$ C grated white onion

1 T Dijon mustard

2 tsp dry Butter Buds

$^1/_4$ rounded tsp sage

$^1/_4$ rounded tsp rosemary

1. Place chicken in a nonstick fry pan and sprinkle with salt.

2. Sprinkle mushrooms over chicken.

3. Place all remaining ingredients in a small bowl; stir until combined and pour over chicken.

4. Cover pan and cook over medium heat for 15 minutes. Remove lid, turn chicken, and cook 15 more minutes, allowing liquid in pan to reduce.

Serve with Wild Rice Medley (p. 130), steamed squash, or fresh spinach pasta.

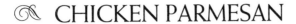 CHICKEN PARMESAN

Total yield: 4 servings
Serving size: 1 half breast
Each serving provides:
Calories: 188
Protein: 29.01 grams
Fat: 4.7 grams
Carbohydrate: 7.4 grams

2 skinless, boneless chicken breasts,
cut into halves

3 T Dijon mustard

1 T white wine

3 T oat bran or polenta

2 T grated Parmesan cheese

1. Preheat oven to 375°F.

2. Rinse chicken breasts and pat dry with paper towel.

3. Combine mustard and wine in a small dish.

4. Combine oat bran or polenta and Parmesan cheese in pie dish.

5. Dip or coat both sides of breasts in mustard/wine mixture.

6. Roll breasts in pie dish mixture, coating both sides.

7. Place on nonstick baking sheet.

8. Bake for 15–20 minutes, or until chicken is cooked.

Serve with Mashed Potato Magic (p. 122) and Simply Wonderful Veggies (p. 136).

⟨⟨ EASY SKILLET CHICKEN

Total yield: 4 servings
Serving size: half breast
Each serving provides:
Calories: 224
Protein: 27.24 grams
Fat: 3.2 grams
Carbohydrate: 21.56 grams

1 C orange juice

2 T honey

2 T minced dried fruit

2 skinless, boneless chicken breasts,
cut into halves

1 tsp cinnamon

$^1/_2$ tsp nutmeg

pinch pepper

1 $^1/_2$ T cornstarch

1 T water

1. In a skillet, combine orange juice, honey, and dried fruit over medium heat.
2. Sprinkle chicken breasts with cinnamon, nutmeg, and pepper.
3. Place chicken in skillet, cover, and simmer 15 minutes.
4. Remove chicken from pan.
5. Dissolve cornstarch in water and pour into skillet.
6. Simmer, stirring frequently, until thick and bubbly.
7. Return chicken to skillet and cook 4 minutes more.

Serve with a double recipe of Quick Carbs for Two (p. 127).

⚬ HERBED CHICKEN

Total yield: 4 servings
Serving size: half breast
Each serving provides:
Calories: 168
Protein: 26.75 grams
Fat: 4.2 grams
Carbohydrate: 5.8 grams

2 skinless, boneless chicken breasts,
cut into halves

¹/₂ C white wine

1 tsp extra virgin olive oil

1 tsp fresh thyme, chopped

2 T fresh mint, chopped

pinch salt

pinch black pepper

1. In a marinating dish, combine all ingredients.

2. Marinate chicken for 4 hours, turning every hour.

3. Preheat oven to broil.

4. Cover bottom of broiler pan with ¹/₄ inch water.

5. Place marinated chicken breasts on broiler rack in pan and broil for 12–15 minutes.

6. Turn chicken breasts; broil for 5 minutes. *(Test chicken by cutting a small slit into the thickest part of the meat; chicken should not be pink.)*

7. Baste with remaining sauce and broil 30 seconds more.

Serve with "Wild-Style" Stuffing (p. 129) or Mashed Potato Magic (p. 122).

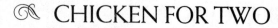 CHICKEN FOR TWO

Total yield: 2 servings
Serving size: half breast
Each serving provides:
Calories: 175
Protein: 27.51 grams
Fat: 3.1 grams
Carbohydrate: 9.27 grams

2 T orange juice concentrate

1 T tamari or lite soy sauce

1 tsp red wine

$^1/_4$ tsp pepper

1 whole, skinless,
boneless chicken breast,
cut in half

1. In a small bowl combine all ingredients, except chicken.

2. Lightly brush chicken with sauce mixture.

3. Cover bottom of broiler pan with $^1/_4$ inch water.

4. Place chicken breasts on broiler rack in pan and broil, 4–5 inches from broiling element, for 10–12 minutes.

5. Turn chicken breasts and broil 5 minutes more.

6. Brush chicken with remaining sauce and broil for 30 seconds more.

Serve with Mashed Potato Magic (p. 122) and a salad.

ENTRÉES

⟨⟨ TERIYAKI CHICKEN

Total yield: 4 servings
Serving size: half breast
Each serving provides:
Calories: 179
Protein: 27.94 grams
Fat: 3.1 grams
Carbohydrate: 9.84 grams

$^1/_3$ C tamari or lite soy sauce

$^1/_3$ C dry cooking sherry

3 T white wine vinegar

3 T water

$^1/_2$ tsp ground ginger

$^1/_4$ tsp garlic powder

2 skinless, boneless chicken breasts,
cut into halves

1. Combine all ingredients, except chicken, in a 2-cup container with lid; shake well.

2. Place chicken in a plastic bag; pour marinade into bag and seal tightly.

3. Place bag in a shallow baking dish and store in refrigerator several hours or overnight.

4. Remove chicken and place on broiling pan, saving remaining marinade to baste.

5. Set oven rack 4–5 inches from broiler; broil chicken until lightly brown.

6. Turn and baste other side of chicken breasts, broiling until lightly brown. Remove chicken from broiler and serve.

Serve with Wild Rice Medley (p. 130).

✍ GLAZED TENDERLOINS WITH BLACKBERRY SAUCE

Total yield: 4 servings
Serving size: half breast
Each serving provides:
Calories: 190
Protein: 26.08 grams
Fat: 1.5 grams
Carbohydrate: 18.05 grams

1 T honey

1 T lite soy sauce

1 T water

1 pound 99 percent fat-free turkey tenderloin breasts
(approximately 2 breasts)

1 1/2 C blackberries

1 T orange juice concentrate

2 T water

2 1/2 tsp cornstarch

1. Preheat oven to broil.

2. In a small dish, mix honey, soy sauce, and 1 T water.

3. Cut breasts in half; wash, rinse, and dry breasts with a paper towel.

4. Brush one side of breasts with honey mixture.

5. Broil 7–9 minutes on top broiler rack.

6. Turn turkey and broil 6 more minutes; baste (use all of sauce during cooking).

7. Slit turkey to check for doneness; meat should not be pink.

8. While turkey is cooking, place blackberries in blender; blend until smooth.

9. Place strainer over a small bowl; pour berries into strainer and strain out seeds.

10. In a saucepan, combine to dissolve orange juice, water, and cornstarch.

11. Add strained berry purée to sauce and cook until thick, bubbly, and glossy.

12. Reduce heat to low.

13. Serve sauce over turkey breasts.

Serve with Wild Rice Medley (p. 130) or Simply Wonderful Veggies (p. 136).

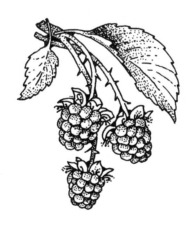

GROUND TURKEY SPAGHETTI SAUCE

Total yield: 6 C
Serving size: 1 C
Each serving provides:
Calories: 133
Protein: 16.33 grams
Fat: 1 gram
Carbohydrate: 14.67 grams

$^3/_4$ pound ground turkey breast, 99 percent fat-free

4 medium cloves garlic, minced

1 medium sweet onion, chopped

1 T fresh basil, minced (or 1 tsp dry)

1 tsp crushed oregano

$^3/_4$ tsp chili powder

2 medium tomatoes, chopped

3 $^1/_2$ C tomato sauce (low sodium and oil free)

1 medium red apple, cored and diced (optional)

1. In a skillet, brown turkey with garlic and onion over medium heat. Stir constantly, being careful not to burn or blacken turkey.

2. Transfer meat mixture (including juice) into a large saucepan. Add remaining ingredients and bring to a medium boil.

3. Reduce to simmer, cooking for $^1/_2$ hour, stirring occasionally. Remove from heat, cover, and let stand for 1 hour.

4. Pour one serving of reheated sauce over a cup of your favorite cooked pasta.

Red apple adds a smooth flavor to this sauce. For a more traditional taste, substitute another tomato for the apple. With pasta, this recipe has 313 total calories and 2.3 total grams fat per serving.

⚛ TURKEY-STUFFED PEPPERS

Total yield: 4 servings
Serving size: 1 pepper
Each serving provides:
Calories: 230
Protein: 26.94 grams
Fat: 5.35 grams
Carbohydrate: 18.52 grams

4 medium green bell peppers

$^3/_4$ pound Turkey Sausage (p. 38)

2 C Basic White Sauce (p. 12)

1 medium tomato, chopped

$^1/_4$ C grated Parmesan cheese

2 C Basic Brown Rice (p. 126)

1. Preheat oven to 350°F.

2. Wash and core peppers. Steam for 20 minutes, cover, and set aside.

3. Brown turkey in nonstick skillet.

4. Prepare 2 C Basic White Sauce (doubling amount on p. 12).

5. In mixing bowl, combine cooked turkey, 1 $^1/_2$ C white sauce (reserve $^1/_2$ C), chopped tomato and 2 T Parmesan cheese (reserve 2 T).

6. Spoon turkey mixture into peppers. Place stuffed peppers into a 2-quart casserole dish.

7. Mix together remaining white sauce and cheese.

8. Spoon mixture over peppers.

9. Bake for 25–35 minutes, or until tender.

10. Serve with brown rice ($^1/_2$ C per serving).*

*If served with brown rice, this recipe has 346 total calories and 6 total grams fat per serving.

ᶜᵏ ITALIAN FISH

Use on 1 pound of your favorite fish. *

Total yield: marinates
  1 pound fish (serves 4)
Serving Size: 1 recipe
Each recipe provides:
Calories: 129
Protein: 0.74 gram
Fat: 2.3 grams
Carbohydrate: 26.34 grams

$^1/_2$ C white wine

1 medium clove garlic, minced

3 T fresh parsley, chopped

$^1/_2$ tsp extra virgin olive oil

$^1/_4$ tsp crushed oregano

$^1/_8$ tsp crushed basil

ᶜᵏ ORIENTAL FISH

Use on 1 lb of your favorite fish *

Total yield: marinates
  1 pound fish (serves 4)
Serving Size: 1 recipe
Each recipe provides:
Calories: 152
Protein: 4.05 grams
Fat: 2.3 grams
Carbohydrate: 28.78 grams

$^1/_4$ C low-sodium tamari or
lite soy sauce

2 T dry cooking sherry

1 T lemon juice

1 T granulated fructose

2 medium cloves garlic, pressed

$^1/_2$ tsp ground ginger

$^1/_2$ tsp extra virgin olive oil

1. For either recipe, combine all ingredients, except fish, in a small bowl and mix well.

2. Pour over fish and marinate for at least 30 minutes.

3. Broil or barbecue fish; use reserve marinade to baste fish during cooking.

Select salmon, snapper, swordfish, halibut, mackerel, or albacore tuna.

⚕ FISH À L'ORANGE

Use on 1 pound of your favorite fish. *

Total yield: marinates 1 pound fish (serves 4)
Serving size: 1 recipe
Each recipe provides:
Calories: 105
Protein: 2.29 grams
Fat: trace
Carbohydrate: 23.06 grams

juice of 3 juice oranges

1 T lime juice

1 $^1/_2$ tsp tarragon

1 tsp dried cilantro

1 tsp ground cumin

1 tsp Dijon mustard

$^1/_2$ tsp dried parsley

1. In a small bowl, whisk together orange juice, lime juice, tarragon, cilantro, and cumin.
2. Pour over fish. Marinate at least 30 minutes.
3. Remove fish from marinade dish and broil.
4. In the meantime, cook remaining marinade in saucepan over medium heat until reduced by half.
5. Remove from heat; stir in mustard and juices from broiled fish.
6. Pour mixture over fish; garnish with parsley and serve.

Select salmon, snapper, swordfish, halibut, mackerel, or albacore tuna.

๏ BREADED FILLETS

Total yield: 4 fillets
Serving size: 1 fillet
Each serving provides:
Calories: 135
Protein: 24.37 grams
Fat: 0.95 gram
Carbohydrate: 7.24 grams

4 (4-ounce) cod fillets*

2 egg whites

2 T cooking sherry or dry red wine

3 T defatted Sona English Style Beef Tea concentrate

$^{1}/_{2}$ lemon

Breading mix:

$^{1}/_{4}$ C oat bran

1 T dry minced onion flakes

2 tsp dry crushed parsley

$^{1}/_{2}$ tsp garlic powder

$^{1}/_{4}$ tsp each tarragon leaves and black pepper

1. Spray skillet with nonstick cooking spray.

2. Place fish in shallow dish; pour egg whites over fish to coat; turn and coat other side.

3. In small dish with a lid, combine breading ingredients; shake well to mix; cover fish completely with mix.

4. Heat skillet over medium-high heat; place breaded fillets in skillet and cook 5–6 minutes; turn fish and cook completely for 5–6 minutes more (slice into fillet to check doneness).

5. Pour sherry and beef concentrate into skillet over fish; bring to boil, then remove from heat. Squeeze lemon over fish and serve.

*Cod may be substituted with flounder, halibut, haddock, or red snapper.

⚘ CRAB-STUFFED ORANGES

Use as a main meal or as a quick lunch.

Total yield: 4 servings
Serving size: 1 orange
Each serving provides:
Calories: 217
Protein: 23.85 grams
Fat: 0.4 gram
Carbohydrate: 29.5 grams

5 large oranges, scrubbed clean

1 C celery, diced

$^1/_2$ C red bell pepper, chopped

$^1/_4$ C green onion, minced

$^1/_4$ C red apple, diced

$^1/_3$ C plain nonfat yogurt

1 T orange juice concentrate

1 T honey

$^1/_2$ tsp celery salt

pinch cinnamon

1 pound cooked crab meat

1. Cut tops off oranges, remove inside fruit meat to bowl and chop finely; chill 4 orange shells and discard the fifth.

2. Cook celery and red pepper in microwave on high for 3–4 minutes, then remove.

3. In a large bowl combine all ingredients, except crab, and toss well; add crab meat and stir until mixed.

4. Remove orange shells from refrigerator and *overstuff* them with crab mixture. Return to refrigerator and chill 45 minutes.

Serve with "Wild-Style" Stuffing (p. 129).

HALIBUT STEAKS WITH WINE SAUCE

Total yield: 4 servings
Serving size: 1 (4 ounce) halibut steak
Each serving provides:
Calories: 166
Protein: 24.34 grams
Fat: 2.1 grams
Carbohydrate: 12.44 grams

4 (4-ounce) halibut steaks

3 T prepared Butter Buds

pepper to taste

Sauce:

$^1/_2$ C diced red onion

1 large clove garlic, minced

$^3/_4$ C low-sodium chicken broth, defatted

2 T flour

$^1/_2$ C plain nonfat yogurt

$^1/_8$ tsp fennel seed (optional)

2 T dry white wine

$^3/_4$ C sliced mushrooms

16–20 fresh asparagus spears

1. Preheat oven to broil; spray bottom of broiling pan with nonstick cooking spray.

2. Saute onions and garlic in nonstick skillet, using 1–2 T of broth as a base to prevent burning.

3. When tender, add remaining broth and bring to a boil.

4. Combine flour, yogurt and fennel seed (for a touch of licorice flavor, if desired); add to skillet and bring to a boil, stirring frequently.

5. Add wine and mushrooms; cook 2–3 minutes.

6. Cover and leave sauce on warm setting.

7. Begin steaming asparagus spears (12–15 minutes).

8. While asparagus steams, place halibut steaks in bottom of prepared broiler pan.

9. Brush fish with prepared Butter Buds and sprinkle with pepper.

10. Broil 5–6 minutes.

11. Turn fish; brush with remaining prepared Butter Buds and pepper.

12. Broil 5 minutes more.

13. Arrange fish steaks and asparagus on serving platter.

14. Pour sauce over fish and serve immediately.

⊗ SHRIMP PRIMAVERA

Total yield: 4 servings
Serving size: ¹/₄ of recipe
Each serving provides:
Calories: 397
Protein: 37.12 grams
Fat: 5.2 grams
Carbohydrate: 50.43 grams

3 tomatoes, peeled and chopped

1 C mushrooms, sliced

¹/₃ C tomato paste

¹/₄ C onion, chopped

¹/₄ C parsley, snipped

2 tsp fresh basil, chopped

1 tsp granulated fructose

¹/₄ tsp salt

dash pepper

1 medium clove garlic, minced

1 pound medium shrimp in shells

1 pound asparagus spears

4 C cooked fettucine noodles, hot (8 ounces dry)

¹/₄ C fresh Parmesan cheese, grated

1. In medium saucepan, combine tomatoes, mushrooms, tomato paste, onion, parsley, basil, fructose, salt, pepper, and garlic.

2. Over low heat, gently boil mixture for 20 minutes, stirring occasionally.

3. Bring water to boil in a separate 2-quart saucepan and add a dash of salt.

4. Shell and devein shrimp; drop into the boiling water.

5. Cook briefly until shrimp turn pink; remove from water and place in sauce.

6. Cover sauce to keep it warm.

7. Steam asparagus until tender; boil and strain fettucine noodles.

8. Place noodles on a serving platter and top with shrimp sauce.

9. Sprinkle with Parmesan cheese.

10. Garnish and serve with steamed asparagus.

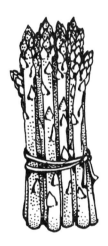

✑ SWEET AND SOUR PRAWNS
WITH COUSCOUS

Total yield: 4 servings
Serving size: ¹/₄ of recipe
Each serving provides:
Calories: 367
Protein: 31.01 grams
Fat: 2 grams
Carbohydrate: 56.24 grams

1 C juice-packed pineapple tidbits
(reserve juice from 20-ounce can)

1 C Jamaican Sweet and Sour Sauce (p. 16)

1 red bell pepper, sliced in thin strips

1 green bell pepper, sliced in thin strips

1 yellow bell pepper, sliced in thin strips

1 pound tiger prawns, raw

1 C couscous

1. Open 20-ounce can of pineapple and reserve juice. Prepare Jamaican Sweet and Sour Sauce using reserved juice and keep warm.

2. Steam peppers for 1–2 minutes and remove from steamer.

3. Shell and devein prawns and cook in steamer basket for 3–4 minutes or until pink; set aside.

4. Bring 1 ¹/₂ C water to boil; stir in couscous. Remove from heat, cover, and let stand 5 minutes; fluff lightly with a fork.

5. Distribute couscous evenly over microwave-safe cooking dish, arrange pepper strips over couscous and top with pineapple.

6. Place dish in microwave; heat at medium setting for 1–2 minutes until warm, then remove. Add prawns and top with sauce; serve immediately.

ENTRÉES

🔊 BETTER BURGERS

Before preparing, see Ground Turkey entry in the glossary, p. 204.

Total yield: 6 patties
Serving size: 1 (4-inch) patty
Each serving provides:
Calories: 112
Protein: 18.8 grams
Fat: 2.6 grams
Carbohydrate: 3.35 grams

1 pound ground turkey, 96 percent fat-free

1/3 C oat bran

1/2 C chopped onion

2 egg whites

2 tsp Worcestershire sauce

1/2 rounded tsp poultry seasoning

1/2 tsp garlic powder

1/4 tsp salt

1. In a large mixing bowl, combine all ingredients.
2. Mix well with fingers and form into 6 patties.
3. Grill or cook in nonstick pan over medium heat, 5 minutes on one side; turn and cook 3–4 minutes more.

Use as hamburger replacer or serve as a side dish for brunch, lunch or dinner.

↻ MUSHROOM AND ONION BURGERS

Before preparing, see Ground Turkey entry in the glossary, p. 204.

Total yield: 5 patties
Serving size: 1 patty
Each serving provides:
Calories: 125
Protein: 24.08 grams
Fat: less than 1 gram
Carbohydrate: 7.28 grams

1 pound ground turkey breast, 99 percent fat-free

1 C chopped onions (reserve $1/2$ C)

4 ounces sliced canned mushrooms, drained

1 large egg white

1 T dry red wine

2 tsp defatted Sona English Style Beef Tea concentrate

$1/2$ tsp garlic powder

$1/2$ tsp crushed sage

$1/2$ tsp poultry seasoning

$1/8$ tsp black pepper

Reserve for frying pan:
$1/2$ C onions

3 T water

1 tsp lite soy sauce

1. In a large bowl, combine all patty ingredients (reserving $^1/_2$ C onions).

2. Mix well with fingers and form into 5 patties.

3. Place patties in nonstick fry pan and cook on medium-high heat, browning one side.

4. Turn patties and add reserved onions, water, and soy sauce to pan.

5. Cover pan with lid and allow to steam cook for 3–5 minutes on medium high.

6. Cut into a patty to ensure doneness.

7. Remove from heat and serve.

Makes a great tasting burger or side meat at any meal.

⚘ CHEESE MEATLOAF

Before preparing, see Ground Turkey entry in the glossary, p. 204.

Total yield: 8 slices
Serving size: 1 (approximately 1-inch) slice
Each serving provides:
Calories: 119
Protein: 19.1 grams
Fat: 1.4 grams
Carbohydrate: 7.5 grams

1 pound ground turkey breast, 99 percent fat-free

1 C 1 percent cottage cheese

1 large egg white

$^3/_4$ C chopped onion

$^1/_2$ C rolled oats

$^1/_4$ C catsup (low-sodium/low-calorie)

1 T prepared mustard

$^1/_4$ rounded tsp salt (optional)

$^1/_8$ tsp pepper

1 T fresh, grated Parmesan cheese

1. Preheat oven to 350°F.
2. In a large bowl, combine all ingredients, except Parmesan cheese. Knead well with fingers to combine.
3. Press into a 8 $^1/_2$-by-4 $^1/_2$-by-2-inch loaf pan.
4. Bake for 20 minutes.
5. Remove from oven and sprinkle Parmesan cheese over top.
6. Return to oven and bake 10 minutes more.
7. Remove and let cool for 20 minutes. Drain off excess oil and serve.

ENTRÉES

⟋ MEET MY MEATLOAF

Before preparing, see Ground Turkey entry in the glossary, p. 204.

Total yield: 9 servings
Serving size: 1 (1-inch) slice
Each serving provides:
Calories: 144
Protein: 12.87 grams
Fat: 3.5 grams
Carbohydrate: 15.25 grams

1 pound ground turkey, 93 percent fat-free

1 C natural salsa or South Border Salsa (p. 10)

1 C tomato juice, salt-free

$^3/_4$ C raw cracked bulgur

2 egg whites

$^1/_2$ C chopped onion

2 T catsup (low-sodium/low-calorie)

1 medium clove garlic, pressed

1 T dried crushed parsley

1 tsp Worcestershire sauce

$^1/_4$ tsp each dried thyme leaves and black pepper

1. Preheat oven to 350°F.

2. In a large bowl, combine all ingredients. Knead well with fingers to combine.

3. Spread into a 9-by-5-by-3-inch loaf pan.

4. Bake 1 hour and 15 minutes. Remove from oven and serve hot.

Serve as a main entree or refrigerate for quick meals and sandwiches.

ENTRÉES

Chapter 8

SWEET SATISFACTION

Sweet Satisfaction

Curried Fruit Compote
Broiled Raspberry Pears
Papaya Bake
Modern Baked Apples
Traditional Baked Apples
Peach Fondue
Crunchy Crumble Topping
Fruit and Grain Crust
Easy Pie Crust
Puff-n-Stuffs
Apple Puff Pie
Fabulous Blackberry Pie
Island Pie
Nonstop Cheesecake
Peach Crisp à la Microwave
Chocolate Pudding
Pumpkin Pudding and Pie
Warm Vanilla Pudding
Chocolate Shakes
Creamy Milkshakes
Hot Spiced Cider
No Kidding! Caramel Corn

✺ CURRIED FRUIT COMPOTE

Total yield: 4 servings or 4 C
Serving size: 1 C
Each serving provides:
Calories: 110
Protein: 3.23 grams
Fat: 0.5 gram
Carbohydrate: 23.15 grams

1 banana, sliced into 1-inch chunks

1 kiwi, peeled and sliced into 8 pieces

1 C strawberries

1 C sliced fresh peaches (or canned, water-packed)

1 C fresh pineapple chunks (or canned, water-packed)

$1/2$ C Creamy Curry Dressing (p. 3)

1. Arrange fruit equally in 4 small dishes and refrigerate.
2. Top each with 2 T Creamy Curry Dressing before serving.

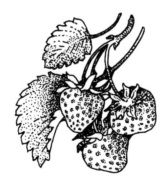

ᘒ BROILED RASPBERRY PEARS

Total yield: 2 servings
Serving size: 2 pear halves
Each serving provides:
Calories: 116
Protein: 0.88 gram
Fat: 0.5 gram
Carbohydrate: 27 grams

2 small pears, fresh or canned in their own juice
$^1/_2$ C partially thawed frozen raspberries
1 $^1/_2$ tsp Grand Marnier*
1 $^1/_2$ tsp granulated fructose
$^1/_2$ tsp cinnamon
2 cardamom seeds

1. Preheat oven to broil.
2. Cut pears in half and remove cores.
3. Place pear halves cut-side up in a 9-inch pie dish, thick ends toward outside of dish.
4. Purée remaining ingredients in blender.
5. Place strainer over a small bowl; pour purée into strainer and strain out seeds.
6. Spoon purée equally over pear halves, reserving $^1/_4$ cup.
7. Place dish 4–5 inches from broiler; broil 7–9 minutes. *Do not burn.* Remove from oven and transfer to two serving dishes.
8. Pour 2 T of reserved purée over each dish.
9. Serve warm.

*Raspberry liqueur or raspberry juice concentrate may be substituted for Grand Marnier.

⟨⟨ PAPAYA BAKE

For that special someone.

Total yield: 2 servings
Serving size: 1 papaya half
Each serving provides:
Calories: 138
Protein: 1.8 grams
Fat: 0.5 gram
Carbohydrate: 31.58 grams

1 ripe papaya

$1/_4$ C orange juice concentrate

cinnamon

2 tsp honey

Suggested garnish: 8 ounces nonfat *frozen* vanilla yogurt (add 80–100 calories/serving)

1. Preheat oven to broil.

2. Cut papaya in half, discarding seeds.

3. Brush each papaya half with 1 T orange juice concentrate.

4. Lightly dust with cinnamon.

5. Place halves on broiler pan, 4–5 inches from broiler.

6. Broil 8–10 minutes, being careful not to blacken fruit.

7. Remove from oven.

8. *For topping:* Drizzle remaining juice concentrate over both halves, drop 1 tsp honey on each, and dust with cinnamon. *Or* spoon 4 ounces frozen yogurt into center, top with 1 T orange juice concentrate, drizzle 1 tsp honey over fruit and yogurt, and dust with cinnamon.

❧ MODERN BAKED APPLES

Total yield: 1 serving
Serving size: 1 apple
Each serving provides:
Calories: 116
Protein: 0.27 gram
Fat: 0.1 gram
Carbohydrate: 28.5 grams

1 Granny Smith apple

1 T natural fruit preserves of choice

1. Core apple, leaving a 1-inch-diameter hole; place in a microwave-safe dish and cover loosely with plastic wrap.

2. Microwave on high for 2 1/2 minutes.

3. Remove apple and fill center with fruit preserves.

4. Return to microwave and cook 10 seconds.

5. Spoon extra juices over apple.

6. Serve warm.

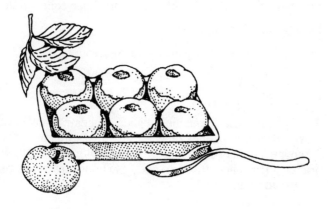

ℛ TRADITIONAL BAKED APPLES

Total yield: 1 serving
Serving size: 1 apple
Each serving provides:
Calories: 146
Protein: 1.05 grams
Fat: 0.4 gram
Carbohydrate: 34.55 grams

1 Granny Smith apple

1 T raisins

1 T apple juice concentrate

1 T natural applesauce

cinnamon

1. Preheat oven to 400°F.

2. Core apple and leave a 1-inch-diameter hole.

3. Drop raisins inside of apple.

4. Combine apple juice and applesauce and fill apple.

5. Sprinkle top with cinnamon.

6. Place apple in baking dish and add 1/4 inch water to bottom. of dish.

7. Loosely cover dish with foil.

8. Bake 35–40 minutes.

9. Serve hot, spooning extra juices over apple.

PEACH FONDUE

Total yield: 36 servings or 2 ¹/₄ C
Serving size: 1 T
Each serving provides:
Calories: 6
Protein: 0.01 gram
Fat: trace (0.5 gram total/recipe)
Carbohydrate: 1.49 grams

1 (16-ounce) can water-packed peach halves

1 T honey

1 T apple juice concentrate

2 tsp cornstarch combined
with 2 tsp cold water

¹/₄ tsp cinnamon

¹/₈ tsp allspice

¹/₂ tsp vanilla extract

1. Place all ingredients, except vanilla, in blender.
2. Blend 20 seconds until *nearly* smooth.
3. Pour mixture into saucepan; cook over medium heat, stirring constantly until mixture thickens and turns glossy.
4. Remove from heat and stir in vanilla.
5. Place mixture into fondue warmer and serve with fresh cubed fruit.

CRUNCHY CRUMBLE TOPPING

Use to top your favorite dessert!

Total yield: 12 servings or ³/₄ C
Serving size: 1 T
Each serving provides:
Calories: 30 (366 total/recipe)
Protein: 1.09 grams
Fat: 0.4 gram (5 grams total/recipe)
Carbohydrate: 5.47 grams

¹/₃ C rolled oats

¹/₃ C oat bran

¹/₄ C polenta

1 tsp cinnamon

2 T diet maple syrup

2 tsp lemon juice

1. In microwave-safe dish, combine oats, oat bran, polenta, and cinnamon.

2. Combine syrup and lemon juice; pour evenly over grain mix.

3. Toss mix to combine.

4. Microwave for 5 minutes on high, stopping after each minute to break up mixture with a fork until it resembles granola.

☙ FRUIT AND GRAIN CRUST

For no-bake pies.

Total yield: 1 pie crust
Serving size: ¹/₈ crust
Each serving provides:
Calories: 75
Protein: 2.63 grams
Fat: 0.2 gram
Carbohydrate: 15.67 grams

1 ¹/₃ C Cream of Rye cereal*

1 ¹/₃ C shredded red apple,
including juice and peel (about 2 medium)

¹/₃ C hot water

pinch salt

1. Preheat oven to 375°F.

2. Spray a 9-inch pie dish with nonstick cooking spray.

3. Combine all ingredients in a mixing bowl.

4. Mix thoroughly with a fork; allow to stand 2 minutes.

5. Press mixture into pie dish, forming a ¹/₂-inch-thick crust.

6. Bake 30 minutes.

7. Allow to cool before using.

*Available at most grocery and health food stores.

❧ EASY PIE CRUST

Total yield: 8 servings
Serving size: ¹/₈ crust
Each serving provides:
Calories: 49
Protein: 18.24 grams
Fat: 0.25 gram
Carbohydrate: 75.2 grams

1 C Fiber One cereal

²/₃ C Shredded Wheat-n-Bran cereal

¹/₄ C Grapenuts cereal

¹/₂ tsp cinnamon

1 tsp granulated fructose

¹/₃ C nonfat milk, at room temperature

¹/₃ C evaporated skimmed milk,
at room temperature

1. Preheat oven to 350°F.

2. In a large bowl, combine cereals, crushing Shredded Wheat-n-Bran until fine.

3. Add cinnamon and fructose; combine.

4. Pour milks over cereals; mix thoroughly and let stand 5 minutes.

5. Pour mixture into 9- or 10-inch pie dish; press and shape into a crust using fork or spoon.

6. To use in recipes calling for *pre-cooked crust* (depending upon recipe, shell may be baked before or after filling is added), bake 12 minutes.

7. Allow to cool.

8. To use in recipes calling for *unbaked crust*, bake according to recipe instructions.

℘ PUFF-N-STUFFS

A puffy pastry treat.

Total yield: 12 servings
Serving size: 1 puff
Each serving provides:
Calories: 45
Protein: 2.58 grams
Fat: 0
Carbohydrate: 8.67 grams

3 egg whites

1 C nonfat milk

1 C unbleached flour

$^1/_8$ tsp salt

1. Preheat oven to 450°F.

2. Spray 12 muffin tins with nonstick cooking spray.

3. In a small mixing bowl, lightly whisk egg whites
   (approximately 20 seconds).

4. Lightly spoon flour into 1 cup measure and level top with
   knife edge.

5. Add flour, milk, and salt to egg whites; lightly whisk to
   combine (batter will be lumpy). Fill prepared muffin tins
   $^1/_2$-full.

6. Bake for 15 minutes, then reduce heat to 325°F; bake for 22
   minutes more. Remove from oven and cool 5 minutes.

7. Slice open tops and fill with your favorite fruit mix,
   applesauce, or Chocolate Pudding (p. 186).

*For brunches or parties: Instead of muffin tins, spray two 9-inch
glass pie dishes with nonstick cooking spray. Pour $^1/_2$ batter into
each pan, covering the bottom. Bake at 450°F for 15 minutes.
Reduce heat to 325°F and continue to bake for 10–12 minutes.
Fill each pan with 2 cups Fancy Fruit Salad (p. 92).*

◎ APPLE PUFF PIE

Total yield: 8 slices
Serving size: 1 slice
Each serving provides:
Calories: 161
Protein: 6.41 grams
Fat: 0.5 gram
Carbohydrate: 32.71 grams

6 large Granny Smith apples, peeled, cored, and sliced thin

$1/2$ C raisins (optional)

5 tsp lemon juice

3 T granulated fructose

$1/2$ C + 1 T whole wheat flour

$1/4$ tsp baking powder

$1/4$ tsp baking soda

1 (12-ounce) can evaporated skimmed milk

3 medium egg whites

2 tsp cinnamon

$1/8$ tsp nutmeg

2 pinches each allspice and white ground pepper

1. Preheat oven to 350°F.

2. Spray 9-inch pie dish with nonstick cooking spray.

3. Place apple slices in prepared dish; sprinkle raisins over apples; sprinkle 2 tsp lemon juice over fruit (reserve 3 tsp).

4. Combine reserved lemon juice and remaining ingredients in blender; blend until smooth; pour mixture over fruit.

5. Bake 50–60 minutes until golden brown. Remove from oven and cool pie on wire rack.

If raisins are omitted, subtract 30 calories/slice. Top with a dollop of Cinnamon Spread (p. 26).

⌘ FABULOUS BLACKBERRY PIE

Total yield: 8 slices
Serving size: 1 slice
Each serving provides:
Calories: 111
Protein: 2.85 grams
Fat: 0.56 gram
Carbohydrate: 23.64 grams

1 baked Easy Pie Crust (p. 179)

1 large ripe banana, sliced thin

cinnamon

3 $1/2$ to 4 C fresh blackberries*

$1/2$ C + 1 T water

2 T cornstarch

2 T granulated fructose (to taste)

1. Fill bottom of pie crust with banana slices.

2. Lightly sprinkle with cinnamon.

3. Place berries in large sauce pan, reserving $1/2$ C for garnish. Mash berries and add fructose.

4. Combine water and cornstarch and mix well. Add to berry mixture.

5. Bring berry mixture to boil over medium heat, stirring. constantly until thick and glossy.

6. Pour mixture over bananas, filling pie crust.

7. Garnish with reserved berries.

8. Chill 3–4 hours. Serve with Warm Vanilla Sauce (p. 24).

Peaches or your favorite berries may be substituted for blackberries.

⟨ ISLAND PIE

Total yield: 8 slices
Serving size: 1 slice
Each serving provides:
Calories: 111
Protein: 3.83 grams
Fat: 0.5 gram
Carbohydrate: 22.8 grams

1 (8-ounce) can pineapple slices, juice packed

2 C (16-ounce) canned sliced peaches, juice packed

1 1/2 envelopes unflavored gelatin

1 baked Easy Pie Crust (p. 179)

2 C blackberries

1 small banana

1. Drain pineapple and peaches, reserving all pineapple juice and enough peach juice to make 1 1/4 C juice.

2. Pour juice into small saucepan and sprinkle gelatin over top.

3. Cook over low heat, stirring frequently, until gelatin dissolves.

4. Chill gelatin mixture until slightly thickened, but not set.

5. Remove from refrigerator and pour 1/4 C over bottom of baked Pie Crust.

6. Cut pineapple rings into quarter sections and arrange over fruit glaze. Top with 1/4 C glaze.

7. Arrange peaches over glaze.

8. Combine blackberries and remaining glaze. Spoon over peaches, leaving a 1-inch border of visible peaches.

9. Chill 3 hours to set. Before serving, slice banana and arrange in a circle on top of berries, leaving a visible border of berries.

◠ NONSTOP CHEESECAKE

If cheesecake is your weakness, don't hold back! Serve plain or garnish with your favorite berries.

Total yield: 8 servings
Serving size: 1 slice
Each serving provides:
Calories: 114 (regular cheesecake = 372)
Protein: 8.18 grams
Fat: 0.33 gram (regular cheesecake = 22 grams)
Carbohydrate: 19.58 grams

1 Easy Pie Crust (p. 179), uncooked

1 envelope unflavored gelatin

3 T granulated fructose

$^1/_4$ C boiling water

1 C plain nonfat yogurt

$^1/_2$ C 1 percent cottage cheese

3 egg whites

$^1/_4$ C nonfat powdered milk

$^1/_2$ medium banana

1 T lemon juice concentrate

1 tsp vanilla extract

$^1/_4$ tsp almond extract

1. Preheat oven to 350°F.

2. Bake pie crust for 5 minutes and allow to cool. Leave oven at 350°.

3. Dissolve gelatin and fructose in boiling water; stir for 5 minutes. Pour into blender and add remaining ingredients; blend thoroughly for 1–2 minutes; pour into cooled pie crust.

4. Bake 1 hour; turn off oven and open door a crack; allow to cool for 1 hour in oven; remove from oven and chill at least 2 hours before serving.

SWEET SATISFACTION

◌ PEACH CRISP
  À LA MICROWAVE

Total yield: 8 servings
Serving size: 1 slice
Each serving provides:
Calories: 95
Protein: 1.03 grams
Fat: 0.5 gram
Carbohydrate: 21.6 grams

4 C fresh peaches, sliced (about 3 pounds)

$^1/_3$ C dried cherries, minced

$^1/_2$ C natural apricot preserves

2 tsp lemon juice concentrate

$^1/_4$ tsp almond extract

pinch nutmeg

3 T flour

1 T ground cornmeal

1. In a large bowl, combine peaches and cherries; set aside.

2. In a small microwave-safe bowl, combine preserves, lemon juice, almond extract, and nutmeg; microwave 20 seconds on high.

3. Remove from microwave and stir.

4. Pour preserve mixture over fruit in bowl.

5. Sprinkle flour and cornmeal over fruit and toss well.

6. Pour mixture into a microwave-safe pie dish and microwave 9 minutes on high, stirring occasionally.

7. Remove and chill to set.*

Before chilling, Crunchy Crumble Topping (p. 177) may be sprinkled over the dish.

❧ CHOCOLATE PUDDING

Total yield: 5 servings or 2 1/2 C
Serving size: 1/2 C
Each serving provides:
Calories: 120
Protein: 4.82
Fat: 1 gram
Carbohydrate: 22.93 grams

2 1/4 C nonfat milk

2 1/2 T cornstarch

3 level T granulated fructose

4 packets Sweet One

1/4 C unsweetened cocoa powder

pinch salt

1/2 tsp vanilla extract

2 tsp dry Butter Buds

1. In a medium saucepan, stir milk and cornstarch until dissolved.

2. Add sugars, cocoa, and salt; cook over medium-high heat 12–15 minutes, *whisking or stirring constantly* to avoid scorching. As pudding thickens, reduce heat to low.

3. Remove from heat; stir in vanilla and Butter Buds.

4. Divide and pour into 5 small serving bowls.

5. Cover with plastic wrap and refrigerate at least 2 hours before serving.

For quicker, burn-free cooking:

1. Dissolve milk and cornstarch.

2. Pour mixture into blender; add sugars, cocoa, and salt; blend 10 seconds.

3. Pour ingredients into a 4-quart microwave-safe deep dish.

4. Cook on high, 6–7 minutes, stirring frequently.

5. Remove from microwave; stir in vanilla and Butter Buds.

6. Divide and pour into 5 small serving bowls.

7. Cover with plastic wrap and refrigerate at least 2 hours before serving.

Serve as pudding or use as a filling for Puff-n-Stuffs (p. 180).

ᏧᎳ PUMPKIN PUDDING AND PIE

Total yield: 6 servings or 8 slices
Serving size: 1 C or 1 slice of pie
Each serving provides:
Calories: 92 or 118/slice
Protein: 6.49 grams or 7.15 grams/slice
Fat: 1.3 grams or 1.55 grams/slice
Carbohydrate: 13.59 grams or 18.86/slice

1 (14-ounce) package soft lowfat tofu

1 $^3/_4$ C canned pumpkin

3 egg whites

2 T granulated fructose

2 T diet maple syrup

2 tsp cinnamon

$^1/_2$ tsp each ground ginger, nutmeg, and allspice

$^1/_4$ tsp salt

1. Preheat oven to 350°F.

2. Spray a 1 $^1/_2$-quart casserole dish with nonstick cooking spray.

3. Drain tofu; place all ingredients in a blender; blend until smooth, 1–2 minutes; pour mixture into prepared casserole dish.

4. Bake 60–65 minutes; allow to cool; cover and chill 2 hours before serving.

For pie:

1. Pour into 9-inch unbaked Easy Pie Crust (p. 179).

2. Bake at 425°F for 20 minutes. Reduce heat to 350°F, bake 45 minutes more.

3. Pie is done when toothpick inserted in center comes out clean. Cool on wire rack.

꩜ WARM VANILLA PUDDING

Total yield: 2 servings
Serving size: 1 C
Each serving provides:
Calories: 149
Protein: 7.49 grams
Fat: 0.7 gram
Carbohydrate: 28.19 grams

2 C nonfat milk

1 1/2 T cornstarch

1 T brown rice flour

1 rounded T raw (turbinado) sugar*

2 T dry Butter Buds

1 3/4 tsp vanilla extract

1. Whisk together milk, cornstarch, and flour; stir until dissolved.

2. Pour mixture into a deep 3-quart microwave-safe casserole dish.

3. Microwave on high for 6 minutes, stirring occasionally.

4. Continue to microwave 5 more minutes, stopping cycle frequently to stir.

5. Remove and whisk in vanilla, Butter Buds, and sugar.

6. Divide into 2 small bowls and serve warm.

*Raw sugar contains nutrients that white sugar lacks. The molasses portion of raw sugar adds a wonderful flavor.

CHOCOLATE SHAKES

Freeze banana slices one day in advance for this one!

Total yield: 2 servings
Serving size: 1 C
Each serving provides:
Calories: 107
Protein: 8.96 grams
Fat: 0.5 gram
Carbohydrate: 16.67 grams

$^3/_4$ C nonfat milk

$^1/_4$ C 1 percent cottage cheese

$^1/_2$ large banana, frozen, sliced into 1-inch pieces

2 packets low-calorie sugar-free instant hot chocolate
(25 calories each)

4–6 ice cubes

1. Combine milk, cottage cheese, cocoa, and banana in blender; blend until smooth.

2. Add ice cubes two at a time, blending on medium setting after each addition until smooth.

3. Divide into two 8-ounce shakes.

᧞ CREAMY MILKSHAKES

Freeze both banana slices and berries one day in advance for this one!

Total yield: 2 servings
Serving size: 1 C
Each serving provides:
Calories: 130
Protein: 9.99 grams
Fat: 0.5 gram
Carbohydrate: 21.39 grams

$^1/_2$ C nonfat milk

$^1/_2$ C 1 percent cottage cheese

1 large frozen banana, sliced into 1-inch pieces

4–5 oz frozen strawberries, quartered
(or your favorite frozen fruit)

3 ice cubes

1. Combine milk and cottage cheese in blender; blend for 15 seconds.

2. Add banana and strawberries *alternately;* after each addition, blend until smooth.

3. Add ice cubes; blend until smooth.

4. Divide into two 8-ounce shakes.

HOT SPICED CIDER

A great evening or holiday warmer.

Total yield: 4 servings
Serving size: 1 C
Each serving provides:
Calories: 103
Protein: 0.74 gram
Fat: 0
Carbohydrate: 25.01 grams

1 large bottle sparkling cider (25 ounces)

1 C water

1 vanilla bean

4 whole cloves

pinch nutmeg

4 cinnamon sticks for garnish

1. In a saucepan, combine all ingredients, except cinnamon sticks.

2. Bring to boil, reduce heat to low; simmer for 15 minutes and strain.

3. Pour into 4 mugs and garnish with cinnamon sticks.

Ꮭ NO KIDDING!
CARAMEL CORN

Total yield: 8 servings
Serving size: 1 C
Each serving provides:
Calories: 39
Protein: 1.4 grams
Fat: 0.3 gram
Carbohydrate: 7.68 grams

2 T evaporated skimmed milk

$^1/_3$ C diet maple syrup

$^1/_4$ tsp vanilla extract

8 cups air-popped popcorn

1. In small saucepan, combine milk and syrup; bring to a boil.

2. Reduce heat to low and cook to soft candy stage (30–40 minutes), stirring occasionally.

3. Remove from heat and stir in vanilla.

4. Spoon over popcorn and mix well.

Use the caramel topping on your favorite desserts or fruit snacks. It has a total of 90 calories and 0 grams fat.

APPENDIX A

Sample Menus ✍

↪ BREAKFAST ↩

- "Bonus" Toast (p. 48)
  Warm natural applesauce
  to top
  Beverage

- New Potato Hash Browns
  (p. 37)
  $1/2$ C 1 percent cottage
  cheese
  Spicy Fruit Kabobs (p. 36)
  Beverage

- Eight-Grain Roll (p. 85)
  Berry Interesting (p. 33)
  Beverage

- 2 slices Bran Bread (p. 59)
  Modern Baked Apple
  (p. 174)
  Beverage

- Hearty Oat Pancakes
  (p. 52)
  Citrus Sauce (p. 20)
  Beverage

- Next-Day Porridge (p. 42)
  8 ounces nonfat or skim
  milk

↪ BRUNCH/LUNCH ↩

- Chicken-n-Broccoli Crepes
  (p. 45)
  Spicy Fruit Kabobs (p. 36)
  Beverage

- Sliced Homecoming Bread
  (p. 80)
  Turkey Sausage (p. 38)
  Basic White Sauce (p. 12)
  Sliced peaches
  Beverage

- Puff-n-Stuffs (p. 180),
  pie-dish prepared
  Fancy Fruit Salad (p. 92)
  for filling
  Nonfat or skim milk

- Breakfast Pudding (p. 39)
  $1/2$ C 1 percent cottage
  cheese
  Beverage

◌ BRUNCH/LUNCH ◌

- New Potato Hash Browns
  (p. 37)
  2 T catsup (low sodium/
  low calorie)
  Turkey Sausage (p. 38)
  Morning Berries! (p. 35)
  Beverage

- Basic Bran Muffins (p. 58)
  Cinnamon Spread (p. 26)
  to top
  Spicy Fruit Kabobs (p. 36)
  Beverage

◌ DINNER ◌

- Glazed Tenderloins with
  Blackberry Sauce (p. 150)
  Spicy Yams (p. 131)
  Small green salad
  Beverage

- Seattle Salad (p. 95)
  Emerald City Soup (p. 105)
  Beverage

- Shrimp Cocktail (p. 117)
  Hot Pasta Salad (p. 93)
  1 slice Onion Bread (p. 82)
  Beverage

- Chicken Parmesan
  (p. 145)
  Steamed mixed vegetables
  1 slice Farmer's French
  Bread (p. 78)
  Beverage

- Stuffed Acorn Squash
  (p. 132)
  $1/2$ C 1 percent cottage
  cheese
  Beverage

- Broiled Barbecued Chicken
  (p. 143)
  Baked Potato Chips
  (p. 121)
  Simply Wonderful Veggies
  (p. 136)
  Beverage

Suggested beverages:
Water flavored with lemon or orange slices or natural,
caffeine-free herbal tea.

APPENDIX B

Substitutions to lower your fat intake 〜

Instead of ...	*Try ...*
Baked goods such as pastries, cakes, crackers, or boxed mixes	Whole grain breads, low in fat
Beef and hamburger	Lean ground turkey; (see Ground Turkey entry in the glossary, p. 204)
Butter	Butter Buds, imitation butter
Butter and oil to saute	Water, broth, nonstick cooking spray
Candy and high-sugar snacks	Fresh fruits, dried fruit leather, sliced vegetables
Canned foods packed in sodium and oil	Water-packed canned foods
Canned fruit packed in syrup	Fresh fruit, water- or juice-packed canned fruit
Catsup (ketchup)	Low-calorie/low-sodium catsup
Cold cereals high in sugar	Sugar-free, whole grain cereal, and hot cereals
Dairy, whole cream cheese or whole fat ricotta	Nonfat Quark, reduced fat or nonfat ricotta

Instead of . . .	*Try . . .*
Whole-fat cheese	1 percent cottage cheese, 1 ounce skimmed mozzarella, 1 T grated Parmesan
Whole milk, 2 percent milk	1 percent skimmed, or nonfat milk
Sour cream	Nonfat or lowfat yogurt mixed with mustard
Whole egg	Two egg whites
Frying	Baking or broiling
Ice cream	Lowfat and nonfat frozen yogurt
Jams, jellies, syrups	Natural applesauce, puréed fruits, natural no-sugar fruit spreads
Metal baking pans and utensils	Nonstick bakeware
Oils—saturated vegetable, coconut, or palm oils, highly processed store oils	For *cold* foods and salads— flax or wheat germ oil; for light cooking and baking below 325°F—*unrefined*, true cold-pressed oils (olive, pumpkin seed, soy, walnut); for baking above 325°F— refined walnut or soy oil
Refined white sugar	Limited amounts of granulated fructose fruit sugar; fruit juice concentrates
Salt	Spices, herbs, pepper, vinegar, low-sodium soy sauce, lowfat/ low-sodium bouillons and broths; limit salt intake

GLOSSARY

Apple juice concentrate (see Sweeteners)

Baking pans (see Pans)

Broth

Beef tea concentrate. A low-calorie, fat-free beef broth sold in a concentrated form. Sona English Style Defatted Beef Tea contains 4 calories per $1^1/_2$ teaspoon serving, and can be diluted with 1 cup of water. Use sparingly, or dilute with twice the amount of water to reduce the sodium amount by half.

Broth, reduced sodium beef or chicken. Conveniently sold in cans, this broth is ready to use in recipes. Excess fat may be "skimmed" from the top by blotting with a paper towel before use.

Bouillon, beef/chicken (cubes or granules). These products are low in fat but high in sodium. When possible, buy low-sodium instant flavor broth sold in boxed form, or dilute bouillon cubes with twice the amount of water. You'll save calories and cut sodium levels by half.

Brown sugar substitute (see Sweeteners)

Bulgur

Available in grocery stores, cracked wheat bulgur is versatile and is used in stews, side dishes, and cereals in this book.

Butter Buds

A brand name of low-calorie powdered butter substitute made from all-natural ingredients. Butter Buds is a fat-free product

used to enhance vegetables, grains, pasta, rice, fish, pancakes, French toast, sauces, etc. This product may be used
dry, in sprinkle form, or *prepared*, in liquid form. Butter Buds
cannot be used for baking or frying because the product does
not contain fat. Butter Buds is one of several butter replacers
available. Other brands may be substituted. (One tablespoon
of dry Butter Buds contains 18 calories and 0 grams of fat.)

Catsup (or ketchup, low-calorie and low-sodium)
This catsup contains one half of the calories and sodium
levels of regular catsup. Usually sold in the diet food section
of grocery stores, it has a remarkable taste and only 8
calories per tablespoon serving.

Cheese
Cottage, 1 percent. Made from cultured skim milk, milk, and
cream. Cottage cheese can be substituted for cheese in many
recipes. It adds a surprising flavor while helping to reduce
the amount of fat normally consumed using cheese products.
A $1/2$ cup serving contains 90 calories and 1 gram of fat.

Parmesan, grated. Parmesan has a strong odor and flavor,
so large amounts are not needed in recipes. Used in small
quantities, Parmesan is a wonderful flavor enhancer and may
help alleviate a cheese craving. One tablespoon contains 33
calories and 1.5 grams of fat.

Cornstarch
A base thickening ingredient. Mix one tablespoon cornstarch
with 6 ounces of cold liquid and stir until smooth. This
mixture can be added to hot liquids as a thickener in the
cooking process. Cornstarch will appear glossy when thick.
One tablespoon contains 29 calories and 0.05 grams of fat.

Couscous
Available in regular and whole wheat varieties. Couscous is
an all-natural quick-cooking grain and traditional dish of
Morocco, Algeria, and Tunisia. Couscous can be found in
most grain and pasta sections of grocery stores, or in most
health food stores.

Defatted broth (see Broth)

Diet maple syrup (see Sweeteners)

Egg whites

Recipes that call for whole eggs (whites and yolks) can be prepared using egg whites alone. Substitute two egg whites for each whole egg. More than 75 percent of the yolk is fat. One yolk contains 250 mg of cholesterol, and more than 5 grams of fat. Egg whites have no fat or cholesterol.

Fats

Fats are the most concentrated form of energy in our daily diet. Fats contain 9 calories per gram. Carbohydrates and protein contain only 4 calories per gram. There are "good" fats and "bad" fats. It is important to distinguish between the two to maintain good health. Fats come from animal and plant sources, and can be divided into three groups: saturated, polyunsaturated, and monounsaturated. *Regardless* of the type of fat (animal or vegetable), all fats contain the same amount of high calories, 9 calories per gram. Fats are differentiated by their chemical structure and by their overall effect on the body.

Saturated fat. Usually solid at room temperature. Saturated fats are found in all animal products such as meats (pork, lamb, beef, etc.), butter, milk, cheese, cream, whole eggs, and yogurt. They are also found in vegetable fats such as coconut oil, cocoa butter, palm oil, and shortening. Because they are *not* water soluble, saturated fats stick together and dry to form plaque deposits. These deposits, along with cholesterol, stick to the walls of arteries and organs. Saturated fats clog arteries, cause cardiovascular disease, and raise blood cholesterol levels. Avoid these fats when possible, and become aware of how food is prepared.

Polyunsaturated fat. Derived from vegetables, nuts, and seeds, these fats are liquid at room temperature. Examples of polyunsaturated oils are corn, safflower, sesame, sunflower, and olive. Polyunsaturated oils have been known to help lower blood cholesterol levels. However, most polyun-saturated oils in stores are specially processed for a long shelf life. This process spoils their basic nature by exposing them to light, heat, or oxygen. As a result, they lack the most nutritional fats important to the body. True unrefined cold-pressed oils are a better choice. They are darker in color than non-cold-pressed or processed oils, and have a stronger taste and smell.

Monounsaturated fat. Liquid oils derived from vegetables. Extra virgin olive oil is the most available oil. It is an unaltered oil and contains a large amount of oleic acid. Oleic acid is used by the body in cell membranes, artery walls, and in skin lubrication.

It is important to supply your body with the *right* types of fat, *essential fatty acids* necessary for normal growth, healthy blood and arteries, skin lubrication and cholesterol break-down. The best sources for these essential fatty acids are flax seeds, walnuts, soybeans, and pumpkin seeds. For cooking, these can be found as unrefined, true cold-pressed oils. Eating cold-water fatty fish such as salmon and mackerel (in 3- to 4-ounce ounce portions) is another way to ingest essential fatty acids and vitamins. The recommended portions of these fish are small, as they are extremely high in cholesterol. Your first choice of fish should be albacore tuna. Remember, fats are deceiving, so it is important to read labels and carefully select and reduce cooking fats to a minimum. It is vital to your health to know the kinds of fat you are consuming and decrease your overall consumption of dietary fats.

Fructose (see Sweeteners)

Fruit juice concentrates (see Sweeteners)

Fruit preserves (see Preserves)

Ground turkey
The following is a nutritional breakdown for each type of ground turkey:

Ground Turkey

% Fat Free	Uncooked Weight	Calories	Protein	Carbo-hydrates	Fat
93	3.5 ounces	140	20 grams	< 1 gram	7 grams
96	3.5 ounces	120	22 grams	< 1 gram	4 grams
99	3.5 ounces	100	24 grams	< 1 gram	1 gram

Reducing the fat content reduces your calorie intake. Fat-reduced meats must be cooked at *lower* than normal temperatures for longer cooking times, as they burn easily. If fat-reduced ground turkey is unavailable to you, ask your butcher to grind your turkey breasts.

Milk

Buttermilk, 1¹/₂ percent milkfat. Originally, buttermilk was the remaining residue from churned butter. Today, it is made from cultured skim milk, nonfat milk, cream, milk solids, and salt. One-half cup contains 60 calories and 2 grams of fat. The 1¹/₂ percent refers to the amount of fat retained to keep flavor and textures. Buttermilk is also available in 1 percent and nonfat forms.

Evaporated skimmed milk. Milk made by removing half of the water from whole milk. The butterfat is reduced to less than one-half of 1 percent. It contains twice the nutrients of skim milk. It is unsweetened and will store 6 months unopened. Cans should be turned every couple of weeks to keep milk solids from settling. One-half cup contains 100 calories and less than 1 gram of fat.

Nonfat milk. Milk that has less than ¹/₂ percent milkfat. It has all the protein and mineral value of whole milk. Because it is nonfat, it lacks the fat-soluble vitamins A, D, E, and K. Vitamins A and D are added. One-half cup contains 43 calories and 0 grams of fat.

Nonfat powdered milk. Air-dried milk. To use, reconstitute and chill in refrigerator for 2 hours for a fresh flavor. One tablespoon contains 16 calories and no fat or cholesterol.

Mustard

Dry. Powdered dry mustard sold in spice section of grocery stores.

Prepared. Mustard in liquid (bottled) form. Made from distilled vinegar, water, mustard seed, salt, turmeric, spices, and natural flavorings. An all-natural product containing 11 calories per tablespoon and 0.7 grams of fat.

Dijon. Also prepared mustard, but with white wine and other spices added. Sometimes sold as white wine mustard. One tablespoon contains 14 calories and 0.9 grams of fat.

Oil (see Fats for additional information)

Olive, extra virgin. Subject to rancidity. Store in refrigerator, and allow to stand at room temperature to return to liquid form before using. A 100 percent fat product. Extra virgin olive oil is a partial source of essential fatty acids required in a daily diet. It is a monounsaturated oil, containing approximately 126 calories per tablespoon or 14 grams of fat. Extra virgin olive oil helps in slowing down the digestive process, creating a longer lasting "full" effect. In this book, however, most of the recipes are oil free. It cannot be used in baking above 325°F. Use a refined walnut or soy oil for cooking temperatures above 325°F.

Orange peel

Dried. Air-dried orange peel, grated fine. Sold in spice section of grocery stores.

Grated. Grated fresh from peel of an orange. Adds citrus taste and smell to recipes.

Pans, nonstick

Suggested pans/tins/sheets for use in the recipes in this book are as follows:

Two baking sheets

Loaf pans: small ($6^1/_2$-by-$4^1/_2$-by-2-inch); medium ($8^1/_2$-by-$4^1/_2$-by-2-inch); large ($9^1/_4$-by-$5^1/_4$-by-3-inch)

Cake pan: 13-by-9-by-2-inch

Pie tins: 9-inch, glass

Muffin tins

Dutch ovens: $4^1/_2$- to 5-quart, 8- to $8^1/_2$-quart

Saucepans: Small, medium, and large

Broiler pan

For baking, nonstick pans are preferred. Since they don't need to be greased, they're great lowfat cooking tools.

Pan spray, nonstick cooking

Helps to keep food from sticking to pans. A preferred nonstick pan spray is a natural 100 percent virgin olive oil spray. One spray adds only 2 calories and 1 gram of fat. Oil sprays contain no salt. This book calls for nonstick pan spray, especially if you do not own nonstick pans. Olive oil spray is used to saute vegetables and ground poultry, flavor and separate pasta, and help cut down on fats normally found in butter, shortening, oils, and other products.

Polenta

Italian cornmeal, found in health food stores and some specialty grocery stores. Cornmeal may be substituted for polenta in the recipes in this book.

Preserves

Fruit. Use all-natural fruit preserves instead of jams and jellies. Natural fruit preserves are lower in calories and are *not* made with sugar. One tablespoon contains 36 calories and 0 grams of fat.

Diet preserves. Use only when necessary. They are extremely low in calories, one tablespoon contains 12 calories and 0 grams of fat. However, they are made with sorbitol and sodium saccharin (which is known to be hazardous to laboratory animals).

Salt

Salt is used in most food processing and preservation. Overuse of salt is a widespread concern. Salt is not a necessary element in all recipes. A skilled use of herbs, spices, and some wine can often replace some or all of the salt called for in a recipe. Salt-free seasonings are widely available. Low-salt and no-salt ingredients are used in the recipes in this book. When possible, use fresh vegetables instead of sodium-laden canned vegetables. When using products packed with salt, drain and rinse food before using. This procedure cuts sodium intake. Use low-salt bouillons and broths. Some recipes call for a pinch or small amount of salt to heighten flavor or regulate yeast growth.

Soy sauce

Lite style. Lite soy sauce has 40 to 50 percent less salt than regular soy sauce. Soy sauce is made from water, wheat, soybeans, salt, lactic acid, and sodium benzoate. One-half teaspoon lite soy sauce contains 2 calories, no fat, and 75–100 mg of sodium.

Sweeteners

Artificial. Artificial sweeteners are widely available. However, many have been found to have numerous side effects. Some studies show an increase in appetite and weight gain associated with the use of certain artificial sweeteners. Although the low calorie content is attractive, caution is advised in using them.

Brown sugar substitute. Artificial sweetener to replace brown sugar. Use sparingly. Sold in grocery stores.

Dextrose. A natural refined sugar. Suggested for occasional use in this book. Sold as Sweet One with Sunette Brand Sweetener in grocery stores. One packet contains 4 calories. Unlike artificial sweeteners, Sweet One holds its taste in baked and cooked foods.

Fructose, granulated. The most suggested sweetener in this book. Fructose is obtained in a separation process from glucose or sucrose. It is the natural sugar found in fruits and is sometimes labeled "fruit sugar." It is 1 $1/2$ times as sweet as refined white sugar, so less is needed in recipes. A caloric sweetener, fructose contains 12 calories per teaspoon. Fructose is preferred as a sweetener since the body does not experience such a rapid rise or fall in blood sugar with its intake.

Fruit juice concentrates. Undiluted concentrates sold in grocery stores in frozen juice sections. Select natural juice concentrates made without added sugar. Concentrates are now available in many flavors (orange, apple, raspberry, pineapple, mixed berry, etc.). Since they are concentrated, juice sweeteners contain approximately 25–30 calories per liquid tablespoon. Store in plastic containers in refrigerator after opening. Keep a variety of your favorites on hand for use in cooking.

Honey. An easily digested natural sweetener. Honey is twice as sweet as sugar so smaller amounts are needed to sweeten foods. A high-calorie food source. One tablespoon contains 64 calories. Use sparingly.

Maple syrup, natural. Slightly lower in calories than honey, maple syrup is the boiled sap of a sugar maple tree.

Maple syrup, diet. An artificial sweetener low in calories. One teaspoon contains only 4 calories. Since it is an artificial sweetener, caution is advised in its use.

Molasses. A thick, sticky syrup, dark in color. Molasses is the residue left from sugar extraction. It has a distinct taste and is a good mineral and vitamin source, high in iron. One tablespoon contains 50 calories.

White cane sugar. Little food value and 12 calories per teaspoon. Sugar is responsible for a rapid rise and fall of blood sugar levels. This rise and fall causes hunger, cravings, and mood swings. Try to reduce your consumption and avoid white sugar when possible.

Turkey (see Ground turkey)

Yeast

A live plant that grows in dough and is fed by sweeteners (see Yeast Breads, p. 75.)

Yogurt

Nonfat, plain. Widely available in grocery stores. Nonfat yogurt is made from cultured nonfat milk, gelatin, modified food starch, and protein. One cup contains approximately 90 calories and no fat. This book uses nonfat yogurt in many recipes. Yogurt can be used to replace sour cream in your daily diet. Plain yogurt can help aid digestion and provide other health benefits. However, commercial yogurt with added sugar tends to inhibit beneficial effects.

Nonfat, frozen. A good ice cream replacer. Nonfat frozen yogurt is usually made with sugar, so 3- to 4-ounce servings are advised. Frozen yogurt can also be made with artificial sweeteners, which should be a secondary choice. Calories will vary depending upon the manufacturer. Frozen yogurt calories are calculated in fluid ounce weights, but the product is sold by net weight.

RESOURCES

Cooper, Wayne. "Wayne's Chicken Soup for Several." Original recipe. Seattle, Washington: 1990.

Dobbins, Bill. "Your Fat Thermostat." *Muscle and Fitness*, October 1990, pp. 117-120.

Dunne, Lavon J. *Nutrition Almanac,* 3rd ed. New York: Nutrition Search, Inc., 1990.

Harter, Jim. ed. *Food and Drink: A Pictorial Archive From Nineteenth-Century Sources.* Rev. 3rd ed. New York: Dover Publications, 1979.

Herzog, Mary Margaret. "Mary's Winter Stew." Adapted from "Please Porridge Soup," *Bon Appétit* magazine, November 1989, p. 221.

Johnston, Linda. "Linda's Meal-in-Itself Rice Pudding," and "Linda's Applesauce Oatmeal Bread." Original recipes. Seattle, Washington: 1990.

Moll, Lucy. "The 'F' Word," *Vegetarian Times*, May 1990, pp. 40-45.

"Nutritional Information for Turkey." *The Turkey Store*, Barron, Wisconsin: Jerome Foods, Inc., 1990.

INDEX

Black beans
  Heartwarming Chili, 106
  Spread, Black Bean, 25
Blackberries
  Fabulous Blackberry Pie, 182
  Glazed Tenderloins with
    Blackberry Sauce, 150–151
  Island Pie, 183
Blueberries
  Berry Interesting, 33
  Hot Citrus Ambrosia, 34
Bonus Toast, 48
Bouillon, 201
Bran Bread, 59
Bran Muffins, Basic, 58
Breaded Fillets, 156
Breads. *See also* Biscuits;
    Cornbreads; Muffins;
    Quick breads; Scones
  Banana Bread, 57
  Bran Bread, 59
  Bran Muffins, Basic, 58
  Eight-Grain Raisin Roll, 85
  Farmer's French Bread, 78–79
  Hint-of-Honey Bread, 60
  Homecoming Cinnamon
    Bread, 80–81
  Linda's Applesauce Oatmeal
    Bread, 65–66
  One-Hour Oat Bread, 69–70
  Onion Bread, 82–83
  Raisin Wheat Treat, 71–72
Breakfast menus, 196
Breakfast Pudding, 39
Broccoli
  Chicken-n-Broccoli Crepes,
    45–46
  Perfect Pasta, 125
  Simply Wonderful Veggies,
    136
Broiled Barbecued Chicken,
    143
Broiled Raspberry Pears, 172
Broth, defined, 201
Brown rice
  Basic Brown Rice, 126
  Breakfast Pudding, 39
  Country Breakfast Rice, 40
  Linda's Meal-in-Itself Rice
    Pudding, 41
  Turkey-Stuffed Peppers, 153

  Wayne's Chicken Soup for
    Several, 112–113
Brown sugar substitute, 208
Brunch menus, 196
Buckwheat flour, Incredible
    Crepes, 44
Bulgur, 201
  Heartwarming Chili, 106
  Meet My Meatloaf, 167
  Next Day Porridge, 42
  Quick Carbs for Two, 127
  Raisin-Orange Pilaf, 128
  "Wild-Style" Stuffing, 129
Burgers
  Better Burgers, 163
  Mushroom and Onion
    Burgers, 164–165
Butter Buds, 201–202
Buttermilk, 205
  Bran Bread, 50
  Creamy Italian Dressing, 4
  French Toast, 49
  One-Hour Oat Bread, 69–70
  Pancakes, Buttermilk, 50
Butter Onions, 133

C

Cabbage, Sweet-Hots Salad, 97
Caramel Corn, No Kidding!, 193
Carrots
  Hearty Stew, 107
  Mary's Winter Stew, 110–111
  Simply Wonderful Veggies,
    136
  Sweet-Hots Salad, 97
Catsup, 202
Celery
  Avant-Garde Albacore, 89
  Chicken Salad, 90
  Chowderhead Soup, 102–103
  Hearty Stew, 107
  Hurry Curry Salad, 94
  Mary's Winter Stew, 110–111
  Seattle Salad, 95
  Shrimp-Atizer Salad, 96
  Simply Wonderful Veggies,
    136
  Wayne's Chicken Soup for
    Several, 112–113

Crepes
  Chicken-n-Broccoli Crepes,
    45–46
  Creamy Berry Filling, 47
  Incredible Crepes, 44
Crisp, Peach à la Microwave, 185
Crunchy Crumble Topping, 177
Cucumbers
  Coldcumber Soup, 101
  Dressing, Cucumber, 6
Curry
  Creamy Curry Dressing, 3
  Dijon Curry Sauce, 15
  Fruit Compote, Curried, 171
  Hurry Curry Salad, 94

D

Desserts. *See also* Chocolate;
    Pies
  Broiled Raspberry Pears, 172
  Creamy Milkshakes, 191
  Creamy Select Sauce, 22
  Crunchy Crumble Topping,
    177
  Curried Fruit Compote, 171
  Easy Pie Crust, 179
  Fruit and Grain Crust, 178
  Natural Fruit Topping, 23
  Nonstop Cheesecake, 184
  Papaya Bake, 173
  Peach Crisp à la Microwave,
    185
  Peach Fondue, 176
  Puff-n-Stuffs, 180
  Traditional Baked Apples, 175
  Warm Vanilla Sauce, 24
Dextrose, 208
Diet preserves, 207
Dijon Curry Sauce, 15
Dijon mustard. *See* Mustard
Dill pickle, Tartar Sauce, 19
Dinner menus, 197
Dip, Fresh Veggie, 8
Dressings. *See also* Salads
  Creamy Curry Dressing, 3
  Creamy Italian Dressing, 4
  Cucumber Dressing, 6
  Honey Mustard Dressing, 5
  Orange Poppy Seed Dressing,
    7

Dried fruit. *See also* Cherries,
    dried; Raisins
  Easy Skillet Chicken, 146
Drop Biscuits, Surprise, 84
Dry mustard, 206
Dry yeast, activating, 75

E

Easy Pie Crust, 179
Easy Skillet Chicken, 146
Eggplant
  Chunky Pasta Sauce, 14
  Mary's Winter Stew, 110–111
Egg whites, 203
Eight-Grain Raisin Roll, 85
Elegance, Chicken, 144
Emerald City Soup, 105
Essential fatty acids, 204
Evaporated skim milk, 205
Exercise, aerobic, xii–xiii

F

Fabulous Blackberry Pie, 182
Fancy Fruit Salad, 92
Farmer's French Bread, 78–79
Fast & Famous Potato Pancakes,
    51
Fats, 203–204
  daily fat intake, xi–xii
  labels showing, xiv–xv
Fish. *See* Seafood
Fish à L'Orange, 155
Flounder, Breaded Fillets, 156
Fondue, Peach, 176
Freezing yeast breads, 76
French Onion Soup, Speedy, 109
French Toast, 49
Fresh Veggie Dip, 8
Fructose, 208–209
Fruit and Grain Crust, 178
Fruit juice concentrates, 209
Fruit preserves, 207

G

Garlic
  Ground Turkey Spaghetti
    Sauce, 152

M

Mackerel
  Fish à L'Orange, 155
  Italian Fish marinade, 154
  Oriental Fish marinade, 154
Maple syrup, 209
Marinades
  Italian Fish marinade, 154
  Oriental Fish marinade, 154
Mary's Winter Stew, 110–111
Mashed Potato Magic, 122–123
Mayonnaise
  Mock Mayo, 28
Meatloaf
  Cheese Meatloaf, 166
  Meet My Meatloaf, 167
Meet My Meatloaf, 167
Microwaving vegetables, 137
Milk, 205–206
Milkshakes
  Chocolate Shakes, 190
  Creamy Milkshakes, 191
Mint
  Herbed Chicken, 147
  Morning Berries, 35
Mock Mayo, 28
Modern Baked Apples, 174
Molasses, 209
Monounsaturated fat, 204
Morning Berries, 35
Muffins. *See also* Scones
  Basic Bran Muffins, 58
  Twisted Apple Muffins, 73–74
Mushrooms
  Chicken Elegance, 144
  Chicken-n-Broccoli Crepes,
    45–46
  Chunky Pasta Sauce, 14
  Cream of Mushroom Soup,
    104
  Halibut Steaks with Wine
    Sauce, 158–159
  Hearty Stew, 107
  Hurry Curry Salad, 94
  Onion and Mushroom
    Burgers, 164–165
  Potatoes Au Gratia, 124
  Seafood Corn Chowder, 108
  Wayne's Chicken Soup for
    Several, 112–113

  Wild Rice Medley, 130
Mustard, 206
  Curry Sauce, Dijon, 15
  Honey Mustard Dressing, 5
  Mock Mayo, 28
Mustard greens, Mary's Winter
  Stew, 110–111
My Best Barbecue Sauce, 17

N

Natural Fruit Topping, 23
New Potato Hash Browns, 37
Next Day Porridge, 42
No Kidding! Caramel Corn, 193
Nonfat milk, 205
Nonfat powdered milk, 206
Nonstick cooking spray, 207
Nonstop Cheesecake, 184
Noodles. *See* Pasta
Nutritional value of foods,
  xiv–xv

O

Oat bran
  Better Burgers, 163
  Breaded Fillets, 156
  Buttermilk Pancakes, 50
  Chicken Parmesan, 145
  Crunchy Crumble Topping,
    177
  Raisin Wheat Treat, 71–72
  Sunday Morning Cereal, 43
Oats
  Cheese Meatloaf, 166
  Country Scones, 61–62
  Crunchy Crumble Topping,
    177
  Hearty Oat Pancakes, 52–53
  Linda's Applesauce Oatmeal
    Bread, 65–66
  Mary's Winter Stew, 110–111
  One-Hour Oat Bread, 69–70
  Sunday Morning Cereal, 43
  Twisted Apple Muffins, 73–74
Oil, 206
Old-Fashioned Cornbread, 67
Olive oil, 206
One-Hour Oat Bread, 69–70

218

Seafood Corn Chowder, 108
Shrimp-Atizer Salad, 96
Simply Wonderful Veggies, 136
Sweet and Sour Prawns with Couscous, 162
Tex Mex Salsa, 11
Wild Rice Medley, 130
"Wild-Style" Stuffing, 129
Red snapper. *See* Snapper
Rice. *See* Brown rice; Wild rice
Ricotta cheese, Creamy Berry Filling, 47
Rising yeast breads, 75–76
Roasted Bell Peppers, 135
Roasted Cinnamon Corn, 134
Rolled oats. *See* Oats

S

Salads. *See also* Dressings
  Avant-Garde Albacore, 89
  Chicken Salad, 90
  Cold Potato Salad, 91
  Fancy Fruit Salad, 92
  Hot Pasta Salad, 93
  Hurry Curry Salad, 94
  Seattle Salad, 95
  Shrimp-Atizer Salad, 96
  Sweet-Hots Salad, 97
Salmon
  Fish à L'Orange, 155
  Italian Fish marinade, 154
  Oriental Fish marinade, 154
  Seattle Salad, 95
Salsas. *See also* Sauces
  Cold Potato Salad, 91
  Heartwarming Chili, 106
  Island Salsa, 9
  Meet My Meatloaf, 167
  South Border Salsa, 10
  Tex Mex Salsa, 11
Salt, 208
Sample menus, 196–197
Saturated fat, 203
Sauces. *See also* Salsas
  Basic White Sauce, 12
  Beef Gravy, 13
  Chunky Pasta Sauce, 14
  Citrus Sauce, 20

Cranberry "Plus" Sauce, 21
Creamy Berry Filling, 47
Creamy Select Sauce, 22
Dijon Curry Sauce, 15
Ground Turkey Spaghetti Sauce, 152
Jamaican Sweet and Sour Sauce, 16
My Best Barbecue Sauce, 17
Natural Fruit Topping, 23
Pinch-Hitting Pesto, 18
Tartar Sauce, 19
Warm Vanilla Sauce, 24
Wine Sauce, 158–159
Sausage, Turkey, 38
Scallions. *See* Green onions
Scallops, Seafood Corn Chowder, 108
Scones
  Country Scones, 61–62
  Sunshine Scones, 63–64
Seafood. *See also* specific types
  Breaded Fillets, 156
  Chowderhead Soup, 102–103
  Corn Chowder, Seafood, 108
  Crab-Stuffed Oranges, 157
  Fish à L'Orange, 155
  Italian Fish marinade, 154
  Oriental Fish marinade, 154
Seattle Salad, 95
Shallots, Island Salsa, 9
Shrimp
  Cocktail, 117
  Primavera, Shrimp, 160–161
  Salad, Shrimp-Atizer, 96
  Sweet and Sour Prawns with Couscous, 162
Simply Wonderful Veggies, 136
Snapper
  Breaded Fillets, 156
  Fish à L'Orange, 155
  Italian Fish marinade, 154
  Oriental Fish marinade, 154
Sona English Style Defatted Beef Tea, 201
Soups
  Chowderhead Soup, 102–103
  Coldcumber Soup, 101
  Cream of Mushroom Soup, 104
  Emerald City Soup, 105

Twisted Apple Muffins, 73–74
Two Easy, 141

V

Vanilla
  Pudding, Warm, 189
  Sauce, Warm, 24
Vegetables. *See also* specific
  vegetables
  Fresh Veggie Dip, 8
  microwaving vegetables, 137
  Simply Wonderful Veggies, 136

W

Warm Vanilla Pudding, 189
Warm Vanilla Sauce, 24
Water, xii
Water chestnuts
  Chicken Salad, 90
  Hurry Curry Salad, 94
  Wayne's Chicken Soup for
    Several, 112–113
Wheat bran
  Basic Bran Muffins, 58
  Bread, Bran, 50
Wheat germ
  Banana Bread, 57
  Next Day Porridge, 42
  Raisin Wheat Treat, 71–72
  Twisted Apple Muffins, 73–74
White cane sugar, 209
White Sauce, Basic, 12
Wild rice
  Medley, Wild Rice, 130
  Seattle Salad, 95
  "Wild-Style" Stuffing, 129
"Wild-Style" Stuffing, 129
Wine Sauce, 158–159

Y

Yams, Spicy, 131
  Yeast, 210
activating yeast, 75
Yeast breads
  activating yeast, 75
  baking tips for, 75–76

Bite-Size Biscuits, 77
cooling, 76
Eight-Grain Raisin Roll, 85
Farmer's French Bread,
  78–79
freezing bread, 76
Homecoming Cinnamon
  Bread, 80–81
kneading, 75
Onion Bread, 82–83
punching dough, 76
rising, 75–76
storing bread, 76
Yellow bell peppers
  Chunky Pasta Sauce, 14
  Heartwarming Chili, 106
  Perfect Pasta, 125
  Sweet and Sour Prawns with
    Couscous, 162
Yogurt, 210
  Avant-Garde Albacore, 89
  Banana Bread, 57
  Basic Bran Muffins, 58
  Black Bean Spread, 25
  Coldcumber Soup, 101
  Country Scones, 61–62
  Crab-Stuffed Oranges, 157
  Creamy Curry Dressing. *See
    also* Dressings
  Creamy Italian Dressing, 4
  Creamy Select Sauce, 22
  Cucumber Dressing, 6
  Fancy Fruit Salad, 92
  Farmer's French Bread, 78–79
  Fresh Veggie Dip, 8
  Hearty Oat Pancakes, 52–53
  Hint-of-Honey Bread, 60
  Honey Mustard Dressing, 5
  Nonstop Cheesecake, 184
  Orange Poppy Seed Dressing,
    7
  Shrimp-Atizer Salad, 96
  Sunshine Scones, 63–64
  Tartar Sauce, 19

Z

Zucchini, Emerald City Soup,
  105